Facilitating Treatment
Adherence in Pain Medicine

Facilitating Treatment Adherence in Pain Medicine

Edited by Martin D. Cheatle, PhD

Center for Studies of Addiction
Department of Psychiatry
Perelman School of Medicine, University of Pennsylvania
Philadelphia, PA

Perry G. Fine, MD

Pain Research Center
Department of Anesthesiology
University of Utah School of Medicine
Salt Lake City, UT

OXFORD
UNIVERSITY PRESS

OXFORD
UNIVERSITY PRESS

Oxford University Press is a department of the University of Oxford. It furthers the University's objective of excellence in research, scholarship, and education by publishing worldwide. Oxford is a registered trade mark of Oxford University Press in the UK and certain other countries.

Published in the United States of America by Oxford University Press
198 Madison Avenue, New York, NY 10016, United States of America.

CIP data is on file at the Library of Congress
ISBN 978–0–19–060007–5

1 3 5 7 9 8 6 4 2
Printed by Webcom, Inc., Canada

CONTENTS

FOREWORD

In 2003, the World Health Organization published the document *Adherence to Long-term Therapies: Evidence for Action.*[1] The issue of adherence was addressed in a number of disease-specific reviews, including, asthma, cancer, depression, palliative care, diabetes, epilepsy, HIV/AIDS, hypertension, tobacco smoking cessation, and tuberculosis. Missing was the area of chronic noncancer pain, which affects approximately 30% of the American population[2] and costs $560 billon to $600 billion per year in the United States.[3] This impressive volume of work by leaders in their various areas of expertise generated a number of "take-home" messages that are particularly salient to the discussion of adherence with regard to pain-related healthcare outcomes:

- "Poor adherence to treatment of chronic disease is a worldwide problem of striking magnitude."
- "The impact of poor adherence grows as the burden of chronic disease grows worldwide."
- "The consequences of poor adherence to long-term therapies are poor health outcomes and increased healthcare costs."
- "Improving adherence also enhances patient safety."
- "Increasing the effectiveness of adherence interventions may have a far greater impact on the health of the population than any improvement in specific medical treatments."
- "Patients need to be supported, not blamed."
- "Health professionals need to be trained in adherence."

These are important guiding principles in any discussion regarding adherence. It is the goal of this book to fill a much-needed educational gap addressing adherence in pain medicine.

We have assembled a highly experienced group of clinicians and researchers to explore the dimensions of "adherence" as it pertains to chronic pain management. We have strived to minimize excessive overlap between certain content areas (chapters) where subject matters converge. But also, we have intentionally included "necessary redundancy"—especially in the domain of psychological approaches to influence adherence—as a means of reinforcing the importance of those (few) tools at our disposal that have been shown to positively influence health-related behaviors.

It is with all sincerity that we express our appreciation to you for "adhering" to your professional commitment to hold your patients' health and well-being in the highest regard by taking what you can from this book and applying it in your day-to-day practice.

Martin D. Cheatle and Perry G. Fine

REFERENCES

1. Sabaté E, ed. *Adherence to Long-Term Therapies: Evidence for Action.* Geneva: World Health Organization; 2003.
2. Tsang AM, Von Korff S, Lee J, Alonso E, et al. Common chronic pain conditions in developed and developing countries: gender and age differences and comorbidity with depression-anxiety disorders. *J Pain.* 2008;9(10):883–891.
3. Institute of Medicine. *Relieving Pain in America: A Blueprint for Transforming Prevention, Care, Education, and Research.* Washington, DC: National Academies Press; 2011.

CONTRIBUTORS

Oscar J. Benitez, PhD
Schatman-Benitez Pain Psychology
  Associates
Bellevue, WA

Lara Dhingra, PhD
MJHS Institute for Innovation in
  Palliative Care
New York, NY

Cristopher Graham
University of Leeds
Leeds Institute of Health Sciences
Leeds, UK

David E. Goodrich, EdD
VA Center for Clinical Management
  Research
VA Ann Arbor Healthcare System
Ann Arbor, MI

**Douglas L. Gourlay, MD,
  FRCPC, FASAM**
Wasser Pain Management Centre
Mount Sinai Hospital
Toronto, Canada

Anthony M. Harrison
Psychology Department
King's College London
Institute of Psychiatry,
  Psychology, & Neuroscience
London, UK

**Howard A. Heit, MD,
  FACP, FASAM**
Department of Medicine
Georgetown University School
  of Medicine
Washington, DC

Robert N. Jamison, PhD
Departments of Anesthesiology
  and Psychiatry
Harvard Medical School
Brigham & Women's Hospital
Boston, MA

E. Amy Janke, PhD
Department of Behavioral and
  Social Sciences
University of the Sciences
Philadelphia, PA

Marc O. Martel, PhD
Department of Anesthesiology
Harvard Medical School
Brigham & Women's Hospital
Boston, MA

Lance M. McCracken
Psychology Department
King's College London
Institute of Psychiatry,
    Psychology, & Neuroscience
INPUT Pain Unit
Guy's and St Thomas' NHS
    Foundation Trust
London, UK

Michael E. Schatman, PhD, CPE
US Pain Foundation
Middletown, CT

Facilitating Treatment Adherence in Pain Medicine

CHAPTER 1

cᐧᐧᐧᐧᐧᐧᐧᐧᐧᐧᐧᐧᐧᐧᐧᐧᐧᐧᐧᐧᐧᐧᐧᐧᐧ

Facilitating Treatment Adherence in Pain Medicine

Adherence—The Great Confounder

MARTIN D. CHEATLE AND PERRY G. FINE

THE EVOLUTION OF ADHERENCE

Dating back to the earliest Western writings about patient behavior, the willingness or ability of patients to follow a recommended treatment plan has been recognized as an important issue—and one that in contemporary times is a major determinant of health-related outcomes. Hippocrates cautioned his contemporaries to "Keep a watch also on the faults of the patients, which often make them lie about the taking of things prescribed. For through not taking disagreeable drinks, purgative or other, they sometimes die."[1] In modern times, healthcare providers continue to be concerned with issues of patient compliance and nonadherence to treatment regimens but often feel ill equipped to influence it. In undergraduate and postgraduate medical education, little is taught about this critical issue.

Surveys of healthcare providers indicate that one of the most distressing features of clinical practices is that of patient nonadherence. Oftentimes the words *compliance* and *adherence* are used interchangeably, but they really do denote very different levels of intent. *Compliance* refers to the extent that patients are obedient to prescriptive instructions of healthcare providers, thus suggesting that *noncompliance* is a volitional act of disobeying salutary recommendations. *Adherence* implies a more active, voluntary, and collaborative involvement of the patient in a mutually acceptable course of behavior to produce a desired preventative or therapeutic result.

The World Health Organization defines *adherence* as "The extent to which a person's behavior taking medication, following a diet, and/or executing lifestyle changes, corresponds with agreed recommendations from a healthcare provider."[2] It was R. B. Haynes[3] who succinctly brought into clear focus the relevance of this clinical construct, stating that "Increasing the effectiveness of adherence interventions may have a far greater impact on the health of the population than any improvement in specific medical treatments."

But through the lens of history and patients' perspectives, there may be unwitting survival benefits of nonadherence. A century ago Chapin[4] commented on the state of medical care at the time, averring, "We might not be surprised that people do not believe all we say, and often fail to take us seriously. If their memories were better they would trust us even less." Iatrogenic complications of treatment and frequency of adverse drug effects continue to be commonplace. And with the advent of the Internet and direct-to-consumer advertising, patients are receiving a barrage of information regarding medical care that can cause skepticism, erode the patient–physician relationship, and increase the rate of nonadherence.

Notwithstanding—but clearly recognizing—these very real concerns, and within the personalized context of each patient's individual circumstances, considerations of adherence must be aligned with and tied to the patient's treatment goals and objectives, self-view and perceptions of quality of life, adjustment to an acute or chronic condition, ability to cope with illness over time, social support systems, and ability to make autonomous decisions. Adherence depends on a strong clinician–patient therapeutic alliance and developing a trusting relationship that is based on collaboration. As the content of this book strives to elucidate this key point, it should also become clear that this necessary therapeutic alliance is far from sufficient to guarantee adherence. Many other factors are determinative, and perhaps predictive, of adherence. But oftentimes, nonadherence can be attributed to a breakdown of the therapeutic relationship, a misunderstanding of instructions from the healthcare provider, or barriers within the healthcare system itself.

INCIDENCE OF NONADHERENCE

Sir William Osler purportedly noted that "The desire to take medicine is perhaps the greatest feature that distinguishes man from animals." (Many texts and journal articles, as well as lay publications, attribute this quote to Osler, but we have not been able to locate original, verifiable source material.) In direct contradistinction, the incidence of nonadherence to medical prescriptive advice is staggering.[5] Up to 50% of patients fail to keep appointments for preventative programs, and 30% to 40% fail to keep appointments for curative regimens. Only 7% of diabetics adhere to all steps considered necessary for good blood sugar control, and up to 60% of patients will discontinue prescription medications prior to being instructed to do so. Up to 70% will not follow medication instructions, and up to 60% will make errors in self-administration, of which 35% of such errors could endanger the patient's health and well-being. The incidence of nonadherence in pain medicine is equally concerning. Over 50% of patients with chronic noncancer pain are nonadherent with their prescribed exercise treatment,[6] and 8% to 62% of patients with chronic noncancer pain are nonadherent to psychopharmacological treatment.[7,8]

There are basic adherence behaviors that promote health and well-being in patients. These include entering into and continuing a treatment program, keeping referral and follow-up appointments, correct use of prescribed medications, following appropriate lifestyle changes, correct performance of home-based therapeutic regimens, and avoidance of health risk behaviors.

FACTORS AFFECTING ADHERENCE

In the field of pain medicine, there are a number of pharmacologic and nonpharmacologic interventions that have been demonstrated to be efficacious in improving pain, functionality, mood, and general quality of life. In a busy clinic where there are often severe constraints on a healthcare

---

Box 1.1

TYPES OF ADHERENCE BEHVAIORS

- Entering into and continuing a treatment program
- Keeping referral and follow-up appointments
- Correct use of prescribed medications
- Following appropriate lifestyle changes
- Correct performance of home-based therapeutic regimens
- Avoidance of health risk behaviors

provider's time and resources, it is critically important to maximize the potential efficacy and overall effectiveness of therapeutic interventions by promoting adherence to prescribed treatments. The consequences of non-adherence in this setting can be dire, including fatalities from accidental overdose involving opioid analgesics with other central nervous system depressant drugs and/or alcohol.

Meichenbaum and Turk[9] outlined a number of factors that can influence the rate of adherence to prescribed interventions. These include patient characteristics, treatment regimen characteristics, features of a patient's underlying disease(s), relationship between the healthcare provider and patient, and the clinical setting.

Patient Variables

There are a number of reasons why patients may consciously opt to not adhere to a prescribed treatment program. These include uncertainty about the efficacy of the treatment, expectations about symptoms, superimposed or intervening illness(es), specific healthcare provider and treatment concerns, past experiences negatively influencing trust with healthcare providers and systems, concerns about long-term adverse effects, inconvenience outweighing potential benefit (i.e., "opportunity cost"), unhealthy attitudes such as pessimism and hopelessness (possibly reflective of depression), competing demands (e.g., financial), and the patient's belief system.

Treatment Variables

Treatment variables that affect adherence include complexity of the therapeutic regimen; how costly, episodically time-consuming, or intrusive the regimen is; and the overall duration of treatment.

Illness and Symptom Variables

Adherence is lowest when treatment recommendations are prophylactic. Although pain is unpleasant, unfortunately in the field of pain medicine the majority of interventions may provide only partial or temporary relief, and there is often a mismatch between what the patient's expectations are for outcomes of treatment versus the healthcare provider's expectations.

Healthcare Provider–Patient Relationship Variables

One of the most important means to improve adherence is strengthening the healthcare provider–patient relationship. When healthcare providers are perceived as hassled, busy, and unapproachable, adherence will decline. Conversely, demonstration of empathy and caring, interest, concern, and availability tend to enhance adherence. Other factors include the level of understanding patients have, including their perception of their participation (or lack of it) in decision-making around their care, and patients' feelings that they are respected. Over the past several decades, demands made on every healthcare provider's time have increased. Concurrently, we have become ever-more technically focused, relying on laboratory or physiological tests and imaging to hone in on mechanisms of disease and improve diagnostic accuracy. Such well-intended motives nevertheless can erode the healthcare provider–patient therapeutic alliance, contributing to diminishing levels of adherence when the patient enters the treatment phase of care. In psychological terms, positive therapeutic transference is difficult to attain with an inanimate object (lab finding, imaging report, etc.).

Organizational/Clinical Setting Variables

A number of factors can promote or sabotage adherence based on organizational/clinical setting structure. These include continuity of care, whether the patient feels his or her care is personalized, the ease of scheduling appointments and referrals, length of waiting time obtaining an appointment, whether there is availability of onsite treatment and diagnostics, staff attitudes toward treatment, and barriers (real or perceived) to access to pain medications or other recommended treatments (e.g., CAM therapies, swim facilities, etc.). Treating healthcare providers need to be aware that adherence is affected by the first interaction with support staff prior to their first interaction with the patient. As well, adherence may be powerfully influenced by circumstances beyond the treating healthcare provider's control once the patient leaves the clinic (e.g., accessibility of pharmacy and pharmacist–patient interactions).

ENHANCING THE PATIENT–HEALTHCARE PROVIDER RELATIONSHIP

There are two prevalent types of healthcare provider–patient relationships: that of an active healthcare provider and a passive patient and that of co-mutually active healthcare provider and patient. A number of studies have demonstrated that when patients feel that they are actively involved in the decision making around their healthcare issues and treatments, adherence increases.[9]

NONPROVIDER ENHANCEMENT OF ADHERENCE

A recent systematic review analyzed the impact of written treatment contracts on adherence involving several clinical areas.[10] The results suggest that the potency of contracts at influencing adherence is weak at best. Although treatment contracts may have some educational and administrative benefits (perhaps more for the provider and facility/institution than for the patient), the evidence to date does not provide compelling evidence for these as a tool that strengthens the therapeutic alliance as a means to promote adherence.

On the other hand, a review of the results of 11 studies evaluated the effect of peer-delivered interventions on recommended treatment adherence in several chronic disease conditions.[11] The authors concluded that peer-to-peer facilitated interventions have an overall positive impact on adherence to medication use and other recommended therapeutic modalities, including exercise.

CONCLUSIONS

What could possibly be more powerful motivators to adhere to an agreed-upon treatment plan than the prospect of reduced pain or, conversely, the risk of a fatal overdose? This rhetorical question could aptly be applied to myriad other highly consequential clinical conditions, especially those that cause immediate and overt suffering, such as asthma or sickle cell crisis or where nonadherence has potentially devastating consequences, such as diabetes management. The fact that adherence seems to be independent of such obvious self-serving rewards makes it a critical factor to understand and all impediments and barriers to optimizing adherence something to emphasize and overcome. Yet there is little formal attention—let alone emphasis—on this obvious but usually unspoken "bridge" that connects a treatment plan to a desired outcome. The purpose of this book is to shine a bright light on this behavioral construct so that clinicians and researchers who are committed to improving the lives of those living with chronic pain and preventing pain-related morbidity and mortality know what they are up against.

We trust that upon digesting the contents of this book, you too will conclude that it is certainly necessary, but far from sufficient, to untangle the web of psycho-neurobiological factors that contribute to the pain experience in order to help people living with pain. Without connecting this marvelous and still-burgeoning science to an understanding of, and reliable means to achieving, adherence, we will continue to fall short in meeting therapeutic objectives.

REFERENCES

1. Hippocrates. *Decorum*.http://www.loebclassics.com/view/hippocrates_cos-decorum/1923/pb_LCL148.271.xml. Accessed May 1, 2016.
2. Sabaté E, ed. *Adherence to Long-Term Therapies: Evidence for Action*. Geneva: World Health Organization; 2003.
3. Haynes RB. Interventions for helping patients to follow prescriptions for medications. *Cochrane Database Syst Rev*. 2001;1:CD000011.
4. Chapin CV. Truth in publicity. *Am J Public Health*. 1915;5(6):493–502.
5. Nieuwlaat R, Wilczynski N, Navarro T, Hobson N, Jeffery R, Keepanasseril A, Agoritsas T, Mistry N, Iorio A, Jack S, Sivaramalingam B, Iserman E, Mustafa RA, Jedraszewski D, Cotoi C, Haynes RB. Interventions for enhancing medication adherence. *Cochrane Database Syst Rev*. 2014;11:CD000011.
6. Alexandre NM, Nordin M, Hiebert R, Campello M. Predictors of compliance with short-term treatment among patients with back pain. *Rev Panam Salud Publica*. 2002;12(2):86–94.
7. Sewitch MJ, Dobkin PL, Bernatsky S, Baron M, Starr M, Cohen M, Fitzcharles MA. Medication non-adherence in women with fibromyalgia. *Rheumatology*. 2004 May;43(5):648–654.
8. Timmerman L, Stronks DL, Groeneweg JG, Huygen FJ. Prevalence and determinants of medication non-adherence in chronic pain patients: a systematic review. *Acta Anaesthesiol. Scand*. 2016;60(4):416–431.
9. Meichenbaum D, Turk DC. *Facilitating Treatment Adherence: A Practitioner's Guide*. New York: Plenum Press; 1987.
10. Bosch-Capblanch X, Abba K, Prictor M, Garner P. Contracts between patients and healthcare practitioners for improving patients' adherence to treatment, prevention and health promotion activities. *Cochrane Database Syst Rev*. 2007;2:CD004808.
11. Enriquez M, Conn VS. Peers as facilitators of medication adherence interventions: a review. *J Prim Care Community Health*. 2016;7(1):44–55.

CHAPTER 2

ᖗᖘ

Treatment Adherence in Chronic Pain

Predictors, Models, and a Role for Psychological Flexibility

ANTHONY M. HARRISON, CHRISTOPHER GRAHAM,
AND LANCE M. McCRACKEN

INTRODUCTION

In virtually any treatment, such as those for chronic pain, certain actions are required by both treatment providers and treatment recipients. The longstanding presumption is that no treatment can be entirely successful without both of these parts in place, although this presumption surprisingly is not always born out in evidence.[1] We refer to an absence in the actions required by the person receiving treatment as "nonadherence." Nonadherence is quite common in general, occurring at a rate of about 50% for prescribed treatments,[2,3] and in chronic pain,[4,5] possibly at a similar rate. Certainly, nonadherence can be dangerous, entails wasted resources, and creates a potential confound in assessing treatment effectiveness.[6] Adherence is an important component of treatment fidelity[7]—without it one cannot say for certain that the treatment is what it is purported to be. These points are important both in clinical and research applications. Finally, current interventions to promote better adherence in general appear too resource intensive and not effective enough.[2,8] So, for these reasons, adherence is worthy of attention.

In the context of chronic pain, there may be unique adherence challenges compared to other conditions. For example, pain treatments are generally not focused on addressing some partially or completely silent underlying pathophysiology, as in the case of antihypertensive, lipid lowering medications, antiepileptics, antiretrovirals, or any number of preventative medications. Rather, pain treatments are generally focused on altering the pain experience and improving function, and therefore these experiences are able to operate as regulators on adherence. This raises the possibility that people can both nonadhere by taking more medication than prescribed (or taking nonprescribed drugs), as well as by taking less, depending on whether or not pain seems out of control, for example. Pain treatments also are rather varied; are used in combinations, including medications, interventional procedures, physical exercise, psychological treatment, educational treatments, and others; and can be provided by teams of providers and not simply a single provider. Adherence, considered broadly, can include taking medications as prescribed, attending treatment sessions, following methods or exercises within or between treatment sessions, applying skills following treatment, sustaining and integrating lifestyle changes, and so forth. Compared to some other conditions, and even among chronic medical conditions, adherence in chronic pain treatment can be highly complex.

In this chapter we take a broad view of adherence, considering it not only in the conventional fashion as "following medical advice."[2] We consider adherence to include all of the elements of required participation of the treatment recipient, either directly instructed or advised, or defined within the methods of treatment provided. A common definition would include the following: "the extent to which a person's behavior—taking medication, following a diet, and/or executing lifestyle changes—corresponds with agreed recommendations from a health care provider."[3] Although the list of adherence behaviors implied here could be long, we focus most on examples of medication adherence and on psychological skills practice and application.

Factors Commonly Associated with Nonadherence

The roots of treatment nonadherence have been intensely studied and appear to be numerous.[6,9] These include patient characteristics and capacities. For example, in this domain, not surprisingly, cognitive impairment predicts nonadherence. Medication specific variables are also important. Here adverse side effects are negatively associated with adherence and simplicity of regimen positively correlated with adherence. Similarly, patient and provider variables may influence adherence, with a better and more supportive quality of interaction with healthcare providers positively associated with adherence.[10] Indeed, psychological variables also appear important. For example, perceptions about medication or disease are commonly found to correlate with adherence, as are levels of distress, acceptance of diagnosis, self-agency/self-efficacy, and others. However, contextual and socioeconomic factors, such as the quality and stability of home, domestic, and social situations also appear to be important.[11,12]

A systematic review by Kardas, Lewek, and Matyjaszczyk[11] included over 700 variables with demonstrated influence on treatment adherence. This wide-ranging result emphasizes the significant diversity of potential factors that may be implicated within any one case of nonadherence to treatment, either seen within healthcare services in general or in pain services in particular. It also highlights a challenge inherent in attempts to create efficient targeted interventions in this area—it raises the question: Where would one begin? We start this chapter by describing current models that are applied to explain (and indeed simplify) how a combination of some, or most, of these variables might result in nonadherence to treatment and from there how this nonadherence might be improved.

Intentional and Unintentional Nonadherence

Although a significant grey area exists between the two categories, adherence can be dichotomized as intentional—the result of an informed and conscious choice to not adhere to a treatment—or unintentional, a passive or nonconscious omission.[13] Intentional nonadherence is thus considered to be a result of a motivated decision-making or evaluative processes. In this area, primarily models referred to as "social cognition"[14,15] have been extended to help make sense of nonadherence, particularly the intentional variety (discussed in later sections). Again, on the surface, unintentional nonadherence does not rely on conscious decision-making processes. As such, it may be considered to result from a "lack of capacity or resources."[16] This lack of capacity comprises problems initiating or maintaining a treatment regimen, which may be explained by memory functioning, disease burden, treatment burden, or simply access to treatments. Such factors may interact; for example, there is a positive correlation between dosage frequency (memory capacity interacting with treatment burden) and medication nonadherence.[13] Indeed, simplifying dosing regimens—for example, using tablets containing combined medications to reduce dose frequency—may improve adherence to medication.[17] Additionally, a poor or inaccurate understanding of one's conditions might also contribute to unintentional nonadherence.[13] Evidence for this is clearly implied in the many studies that show that beliefs about illness and medication can predict adherence behavior.[18] Finally, the quality of the relationship between the patient and the clinician(s) can also influence unintentional treatment nonadherence,[13] as mentioned briefly earlier. Studies demonstrate that faith in the patient's respective physician, number of physician visits, and provision of information can promote adherence.[19-21] Interventions for unintentional nonadherence might involve simplifying medication regimens, introducing memory aides, improving faith or trust in the provider, or providing information about treatment of the disease.

Dichotomizing treatment nonadherence into intentional and unintentional categories offers a pragmatic way to conceptualize the problem. This can allow a clinician to rapidly generate methods to intervene, based on motivational models (discussed in later sections) or the patient, treatment, and patient–provider factors identified here. However, in reality these categories overlap considerably. For example, while a misunderstanding of the condition or treatment may make nonadherence more likely, based on this factor alone, nonadherence to medication is still a motivated choice, albeit one made based on a poor understanding. Further, while a true deficit in memory appears to be the clearest example of unintentional nonadherence, Molloy et al.[16] muddy even these ostensibly clear waters by suggesting that forgetting is more likely when motivation to take medication is low.

COMMON MODELS OF ADHERENCE

Cognitive psychologists have long been interested in the role of decision-making processes in explaining treatment nonadherence. Given the primary role of motivation in each model, most may be presumed to relate more to intentional than unintentional nonadherence. Several well-researched models now exist. Three of these are "social-cognition" models, which are briefly outlined in this chapter. In addition, we describe a newer health behavior change model, the Capability, Opportunity and Motivational Model of Behavior that aims to synthesize the aforementioned models.

Social-Cognition Models: Theory of Planned Behavior

The Theory of Planned Behavior[14] posits a linear sequence of cognitive processes that result in a behavior, in this case adherence to treatment. Here the most proximal influence on the behavior in question (i.e., adherence) is one's *intention* to enact the behavior. This intention is in turn informed by (a) one's attitudes toward that behavior—the extent to which the behavior is positively or negatively valued; (b) a subjective norm regarding the perceived social value of the behavior, or the pressure society exerts on the person to engage in the behavior; and (c) perceived behavioral control—one's perceptions of one's own ability to perform the behavior.

A meta-analyses of 27 studies[22] investigated the extent to which features of this model predicted adherence to a range of treatments (medication, exercise, and dietary advice) in a range of chronic diseases (e.g., HIV, epilepsy, and COPD). Results here indicated that intention had a small to medium magnitude of influence on adherence behavior. In addition, the more distal variables in the model predicted very modest amounts of variance (9%). This suggests this model has limited predictive, or explanatory, value for guiding the development of adherence interventions, perhaps reflecting what is commonly referred to as a significant "intention–behavior gap."[22]

There are several possible reasons for the modest level of explanation achieved with the Theory of Planned Behavior. Influential socioeconomic variables, such as access to treatment, are not considered nor are emotional processes. Indeed, low mood is an incremental and robust negative predictor of adherence to HIV medication, for example.[23] Given the centrality of physical symptoms in chronic pain, it is perhaps no surprise that in a multicenter study intentions were found to have no significant predictive value for adherence to multidisciplinary pain treatment.[24]

Leventhal's Self-Regulatory Model

Leventhal's Self-Regulatory Model[15] assumes that patients are active problem-solvers, who are motivated to make sense of health threats. The Self-Regulatory Model thus suggests that adherence behaviors are predicted by the results of this evaluative process, referred to as an illness representation. An illness representation is a multidimensional framework of beliefs regarding a symptom or health threat, including how long it will last, the consequences, and, importantly, whether the illness or symptom(s) can be controlled by treatment or one's own behavior. In contrast to the Theory of Planned Behavior, this model incorporates a feedback loop, such that the success or failure of a treatment, or coping method, subsequently updates the illness representation.

A meta-analysis of 23 studies investigated the predictive value of this model for adherence to medication, exercise, and diet recommendations.[25]

This analysis found that illness representations were very weak predictors of adherence behaviors, perhaps to an even lesser extent than components of the Theory of Planned Behavior. This model could be criticized as not taking account of the many motivations that lie outside of disease self-management, including one's overarching values[26] and socioeconomic circumstances. Indeed, adherence may be better predicted by cognitions that are more proximal to an adherence behavior, such as a patient's beliefs about his or her medication. This is addressed by another explanatory model—the Necessity Concerns Framework.

Necessity Concerns Framework

The Necessity-Concerns Framework[27,28] proposes that patients weigh the benefits of treatment against its perceived costs. The result of this process is a decision to adhere to treatment recommendations or act otherwise. Aspects of this simple evaluation can be measured with a purpose-built questionnaire, the Beliefs about Medicines Questionnaire.[29] This has two subscales, Necessity (i.e., the benefits of treatment) and Concerns (e.g., fears about side effects). A recent meta-analysis of this measure (94 studies) found that both necessity and concerns have some, albeit limited, ability to explain adherence to treatment.[30] In line with the preceding models, similar criticisms have been raised about this model, including that it includes little consideration of socioeconomic context, patient–provider variables, or other automatic processes such as emotions or habit.

Interventions Derived from Social-Cognition Models

Given the relatively narrow focus and limited explanatory power provided by each model, it is perhaps not surprising that cognitive-behavioral interventions informed by these models show limited efficacy[8]—at best resulting in a combined small effect on outcomes.[31] Nonetheless, we briefly describe examples of adherence interventions based on the preceding models.

Brown and colleagues[32] randomized people with epilepsy to a treatment as usual control group or an intervention group receiving an "implementation intentions" worksheet, derived from the Theory of Planned Behavior. This worksheet contained "if-then" statements that encouraged patients to consider in advance where and when they would take their medication, alongside reminding them of how important it is to take medication. This resulted in a comparative significant improvement in the number of pre-scribed doses taken and the number taken on schedule.

Petrie and colleagues[12] trialed a text-message intervention to improve adherence to asthma prevention medication. This targeted the processes described in Leventhal's Self-Regulatory Model and also the Necessity Concerns Framework, by texting participants messages designed to change their illness representation and/or medication beliefs. Here participants were sent roughly one text a day for 18 weeks. This intervention resulted in a statistically significant 10% average improvement in adherence.

Perhaps the mostly widely-used intervention to improve treatment adherence is motivational interviewing, which targets the basic volitional process implicit in all the described models. Motivational interviewing enacts four principles, including: 1) Expressing empathy, actively listening to the patients perspective, without blaming or judgement; 2) Developing discrepancy, helping patients see the gap between their personal goals and present behavior (i.e. adherence behaviors); 3) Rolling with resistance, reflecting and rephrasing patients arguments against change instead of pushing against resistance; and 4) Supporting self-efficacy using language which demonstrates belief in the patient's ability to make changes.[33] Motivational Interviewing has been applied with some success to improve adherence to medication for HIV, hypertension, and diabetes, amongst other conditions.[31]

Composite Model: The Capability, Opportunity, and Motivation Model of Behavior

The COM-B[34] is a broad framework which was designed to address the aforementioned limitations of earlier models. COM-B incorporates the main tenets of each, and adds variables that may lie outside of motivational processes (for example, those relating to unintentional non-adherence). It classifies a broad range of variables into three interdependent categories that can influence a given behavior (i.e. adherence), including: 1) Capability, the capacity to engage in the behavior; 2) Opportunity, contextual factors which lie outside of the individual that enable or prompt the behavior; 3) Motivation, involving volitional processes which are reflective (evalua-tive processes, such as those implicit in the previous models) or automatic (emotions and impulses).[35]

COM-B is a newer model. It has been heralded as particularly appropri-ate for medication non-adherence.[35] This is principally because it appro-priately includes a range of variables that may explain intentional or unintentional treatment non-adherence (or the grey area between these categories). This is clinically useful because it encourages treatment providers to think about a broad range of factors that may influence adherence. A patient may not adhere for any number of reasons, which may be motivational (e.g. linked to beliefs about medication), contextual (poor access to high cost treatment) or related to capability (e.g., cognitive functioning).

However, the apparent strength of the COM-B model is the breadth of factors that it appears to accommodate, which may also reflect a weakness. Although this model can help us to understand what might contribute to non-adherence it lacks a coherent theoretical delineation of how variables interact to result in non-adherence. Put another way, its greater focus on factors and methods means there is less of a focus on key principles and processes. Thus, it offers limited guidance in formulating non-adherence to treatment in a given case or group of cases. Indeed, one could argue that COM-B is not a model per se, but rather a broader framework or method of categorization. Nonetheless, compared to its predecessors it does come closer to providing a more accurate illustration of a range of factors that may influence adherence. COM-B links to a method of behavior change, the Behavior Change Wheel.[34] This again outlines a diverse range of intervention methods which can be used to change behavior. Similarly, this is useful in considering the range of tools at one's disposal, but the same caveats regarding integrating tools to build a coherent intervention also applies.

MEDICATION ADHERENCE IN PAIN MANAGEMENT

As noted earlier, it has been quite common for many years to estimate rates of non-adherence for those using long-term medications at 50%.[6,9] However, in studies of people with chronic pain we find varying rates of adherence depending how the question is phrased and the population studied. In specialty pain treatment centers in the UK 63.5% reported that they took their medication exactly as instructed, yielding a non-adherence rate of 36.5%. However, within this latter group, 57.1% reported missing doses, and a remarkable 74.9% reported taking more frequent, or higher, doses than prescribed.[36] In a primary care context, also in the UK, responses to the same questions yielded different percentages of non-adherence, including 24.4%, 52.0% and 30.4%, respectively.[37] In these studies, as a general summary, based on analyses of predictors of use patterns, both non-adherence and underuse were predicted by concerns about effects of medications, and overuse was predicted by perceived need for the medication. Without it having been expected, concerns experienced while taking medications for pain appeared to contribute to greater depression and disability, suggesting that the taking of medications for pain carries the potential (via these concerns) for additional distress and functional impacts in those already suffering from the condition itself.[36] A study from Belgium showed somewhat lower rates of underuse and overuse, 34% and 14%,[38] and the basis for these differences seems to arise from a more selective definition of these aspects of nonadherence.

A systematic review of studies on medication adherence in people with chronic pain included 14 studies.[4] The authors summarized non-adherence as ranging from 7.7% to 52.9%, underuse at 29.9% and overuse at 13.7%. It is notable, however, that their definitions of non-adherence, overuse, and under use, were based on operational definitions in the studies reviewed and were relatively conservative, including such criteria as patterns of repeated abuse, or misuse, or based on urine screen results. In the earlier studies in the UK, if the patient said they took more or less than prescribed, this was regarded as non-adherence. Besides studies investigating adherence rates, Broekmans and colleagues[4] were unable to make clear statements about relations between adherence and clinical outcome due to the limited number of studies and methodological limitations in those identified. In addition, they averred that no reported studies investigated variables that might influence adherence or the types of interventions that might most effectively enhance adherence. This final part of their conclusion is consistent with the findings of a systematic review of psychosocial predictors of nonadherence to chronic medication by Zwikker et al.[9] From their examination of 30 studies, they concluded that "results do not provide psychosocial targets for the developments of new interventions in clinical practice."

A recent Cochrane review assessed the effects of interventions to enhance adherence to medications.[8] It included 182 randomized control trials (RCTs) with heterogeneous medical problems, medications, adherence interventions, and outcome measures. Seventeen studies with the lowest risk of bias included complex interventions, typically delivered by allied healthcare providers such as pharmacists. Only five studies reported improvements in both adherence and clinical outcomes. The interventions were highly varied, and even the most effective generally produced small effects.[8] Most of the included studies focused on asthma, coronary artery disease, diabetes, and HIV. There were trials in postsurgical pain and in rheumatoid arthritis, but medications for chronic pain were not a focus in any of the studies. An additional recent review found that, based on six studies across a range of varying medical conditions, combinations of motivational interviewing and cognitive-behavioral methods may hold promise for promoting better medication adherence, although four of the studies were cohort designs and only one an RCT.[39]

Adherence to Skills Training in Pain Management

As mentioned, adherence is a long-standing interest in pain management, particularly within approaches that frame pain as a problem requiring behavior change and self-management. In part, attention to adherence has been regarded as a way to reduce high rates of relapse following initially successful treatment.[5] The assumption has been that people with chronic pain need to learn new skills, abandon unhelpful strategies, and persist with the use of their new skills to maintain the benefits they may have gained.[40] The evidence surrounding this assumption suggests resolution to this problem is not straightforward.

In a large-scale clinical study (N = 2,435), based in an intensive, interdisciplinary pain management center, a measure of adherence to exercise, stretching, pacing, and cognitive restructuring at a one-month follow-up period was examined in relation to psychological well-being during the follow-up interval.[40] Here it was found that the skills trained in treatment appeared to be used at moderate rates, with pacing, thought challenging, stretching, and exercise used at least five days per week by 66.8%, 46.4%, 74.4%, and 59.6% of participants, respectively. It was also found that adherence to the skills significantly predicted psychological well-being, but adherence accounted for only a very small amount of variance in this outcome, namely less than 3% for adherence combined, suggesting that adherence in this situation provided little perceived benefit. The authors concluded that their findings "question the emphasis normally given to adherence in the maintenance of cognitive and behavioral change" in treatment for chronic pain.[40]

In a subsequent study, also based in an intensive pain management setting (N = 567), adherence to seven strategies was measured based on daily records that were routinely checked by staff.[41] The seven strategies included activity pacing, using a flare-up plan, stretching, desensitization, thought challenging, fitness exercises, and goal-setting. Two of these, flare-up plans and fitness exercises, were not used in subsequent analyses. As for the five strategies examined, adherence appeared on par with other rates discussed here with 50.6% of participants using four of five of the strategies on a consistent basis. In their further analyses, the authors found that practicing four or five out of the five strategies on a consistent basis was associated with improvements in pain, disability, and depression at posttreatment. Remarkably, these relations remained significant in analyses where baseline levels of self-efficacy, catastrophizing, and fear-avoidance beliefs were controlled. One key difference from the study of Curran and colleagues,[40] in addition to the measures of outcome and adherence, is that Curran and colleagues examined adherence at follow-up and Nicholas and colleagues[41] examined adherence during treatment.

A recent study that raised the question "Can we improve engagement and adherence in cognitive-behavioral therapy (CBT) for chronic back pain?" seems to indicate that we cannot.[42] Here a tailored version of CBT, including learning preferences of the participants, was no better at creating engagement and adherence than standard therapy in terms of session attendance or ratings of adherence to recommended coping skills practice. These researchers did find that number of sessions attended and adherence ratings across the two conditions were correlated with improvements in disability, goal achievement, and satisfaction, although these correlations overall were small.

Psychological Flexibility: An Organizing Framework

A relatively new approach that could improve our understanding of treatment adherence is the Psychological Flexibility (PF) Model, the model underlying Acceptance and Commitment Therapy (ACT).[43] ACT is a form of CBT,[44] one of the so-called "third-wave" or "mindfulness-based" psychological treatments. It was developed to address common problems with health and human performance, broadly considered, and appeared in a first full book-length description in the late 1990s.[43] Since that time, evidence supporting the application of ACT has grown rapidly in the context of behavioral medicine,[45] and in recent years this approach has gained support in the treatment of chronic pain[46,47] and a wide range of other conditions.[48-51]

An important feature of ACT includes its underpinnings in the PF Model. Layered on this foundation are the parallel developments that are associated with ACT, including a theory of language and cognition, which have been in development for more than 20 years,[52,53] its underlying philosophy(referred to as functional contextualism), and its combined program of basic and applied research(referred to as contextual behavioral science).[54]

What Is Psychological Flexibility?

Psychological flexibility has been defined as the capacity for an individual to persist with or change behavior in a manner that includes conscious and open contact with thoughts and feelings, appreciates what situations afford, and serves one's goals and values.[55] Certainly the elements of "capacity to persist" and "serves one's goals" found in this model carry direct applicability to adherence. A model that shows the elements of PF is presented in Figure 2.1. It incorporates six integrated processes, including acceptance, defusion, self-as-context, present moment awareness, values, and committed action.[43,44]

In short, *acceptance* reflects an individual's willing engagement in activities in a way that includes contact with unwanted thoughts and feelings or other experiences, without defense or attempts to struggle with or control them, when to do so serves one's goals.[47] *Cognitive defusion* refers to one's ability to experience a distinction between thoughts and the objects, events, or people they describe. It also involves contacting these private experiences but at the same time not being overly dominated by the meaning and influences carried in them to the exclusion of other direct experience.[54] *Self-as-observer* is the person's ability to take a particular stance or perspective or hold a sense-of-self, where the person is aware of his or her thoughts and feelings but not attached to them as a matter of identity or harmed by them.[47,56] *Present-moment awareness*, or attention, is the ability to maintain contact with direct experiences moment to moment and is akin to the qualities cultivated in mindfulness meditation.[57] *Values* are life directions, or freely chosen qualities of action the person defines as

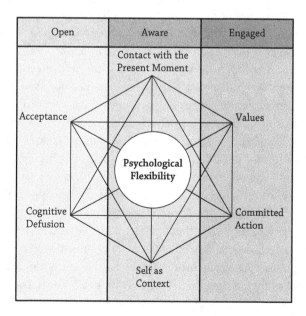

Figure 2.1. ACT's Psychological Flexibility Model, both six-part and three-part.

important. Distinct from goals, values are not obtainable as an objective but rather can be worked toward moment by moment.[44] Importantly, values can feed into goals. Last, *committed action* can be thought of as the person's active choosing and rechoosing to flexibility persist in a particular course of action based on his or her values and goals in a way that can meet barriers and continue, allow for failure and discomfort, but also change in a course of action if shown to be unhelpful.[58]

Taken together, the four processes on the left side of Figure 2.1 amount to mindfulness and acceptance processes and values and committed action; those on the right reflect more commitment and behavior change processes.[54] Put another way, people's patterns of behavior might be described as "psychologically inflexible" if they attempt to avoid unwanted experiences and this results in failures in reaching goals; if they are overwhelmed and guided exclusively in their thoughts and cannot assume a perspective separate from thoughts and feelings; if they have a preoccupation with the past or future; if they have little sense of their values and do not pursue them; if they persist in actions even when these do not achieve their goals; or if they engage in behavior on impulse, excessively influenced by transient thoughts or feelings. As seen in Figure 2.1, the PF Model can be further distilled into three broader processes, known as Open, Aware, and Engaged.[59,60]

The PF Model provides a comprehensive organizing conceptual framework that may apply to a variety of treatment-related nonadherence problems. Unlike previously described alternative cognitive or transtheoretical models, one advantage of PF is that it more fully integrates cognitive, motivational, and functional dimensions of behavior.[47] The PF Model is distinct from cognitive or transtheoretical models in several important ways, which may translate to the development of novel treatment methods. Previous adherence theories and associated treatments usually assume a person needs to (a) build confidence, or enhance self-efficacy, in order to successfully execute a given adherence behavior (e.g., taking prescribed medication, attending treatment sessions, learning and using skills); (b) feel less depressed and more optimistic to perform adherence behavior; (c) know, or understand, why adherence is important (with an emphasis on disease education); or (d) influence, change, or directly challenge mistaken beliefs about disease and treatments. Another important tacit assumption in other adherence behavior models is that a person must adhere in order to be well and healthy. Psychological flexibility does not assume these are required.

In contrast to other conventional models, the PF Model assumes that effective action, including adherence behavior, can occur in the presence of contrary or disturbing thoughts or feelings or a lack of confidence. Rather than changing the content, frequency, or intensity of feelings or beliefs about a disease or treatments, or challenging thoughts directly, ACT is principally concerned with helping people experience a decreased influence from thoughts, feelings, or beliefs so that they can align their behavior with the goal at hand. ACT uses experiential exercises, including metaphorical language, paradoxes, and stories introduced by the therapist, that aim to help people come into contact with psychological processes more directly and help them learn to relate to their thoughts and feelings in a way that produces better outcomes.[54]

Although ACT does not seek to convince or persuade, it does bring into focus the question of how effective or "workable" a person's behavior is by repeatedly setting it against the things he or she most values in life (e.g., performing as a caring parent, acting with honesty, devotion to work, etc.). The emphasis on values and workability provides a useful framework to enhance clarity of an individual's informed choices in treatment, which in combination with available medical advice may allow the person to more fully consider either following, or not following, prescriptions. This may be especially helpful when treatments come with serious risks, overwhelming side effects, or potentially limited therapeutic impact. In some circumstances, a choice to not engage with treatment will result in increased symptoms but may allow the person to actually function better. Conversely, ACT's specifically pragmatic focus may also help in the context of problems that are different from and collateral to pain, such as hypertension or obvious symptoms that do not appear until the onset of more serious health events as a result of nonadherence.

In addition to processes within ACT that are specifically focused on goals and persistent engagement, and in dealing effectively to barriers to this engagement, ACT can also support therapeutic relationships that are particularly consistent with greater adherence. ACT shares features with motivational interviewing in that it emphasizes a focus on therapeutic interactions that create helpful change rather than unwittingly keeping people stuck.[61] ACT includes a therapeutic stance that is equal, compassionate, focused on patient goals, and noncoercive. These features are likely to model the same processes and carry precisely the same influences as particular strategies within motivational interviewing (MI), such as the use of empathy, highlighting discrepancies, and "rolling with resistance."

Examples of Adherence-Related Studies of ACT

At present there are at least five separate examples of areas where ACT has been applied to adherence-related problems. Two studies in the literature investigate ACT in the context of adherence to medical treatment specifically, though neither of these were studies of chronic pain. One unpublished RCT aimed to improve men's attendance to an erectile rehabilitation program, which comprises intracavernosal injection therapy after radical prostatectomy, using seven sessions of ACT compared to enhanced monitoring.[62] The second was an uncontrolled pilot study to explore whether a three- to five-week ACT group program improved adherence to highly active antiretroviral therapy in people with HIV.[63] Both studies showed promising trends of improvement in adherence-related outcomes. Nelson and colleagues[62] showed significantly higher numbers of penile injections per week (verified by syringe count) and greater satisfaction with treatment compared to enhanced monitoring at four and eight months.

Moitra et al.[63] observed reductions in viral load count and increases in CD4 lymphocytes in HIV at posttreatment in their trial of ACT. What is striking about this HIV study in particular is that the sample was drawn from an urban, minority, low-socioeconomic community in the United States, which ordinarily would be considered a hard-to-reach population. One limitation of both of these medication adherence studies is that neither directly examined the relationship between PF processes and adherence measures at pre- and posttreatment. In fact, currently there are no direct studies examining whether PF processes represent important determinants of either self-reported adherence or more objective measures of adherence behavior or whether both adherence and these processes independently contribute to health and well-being. A helpful next step in this area could be to examine the role of PF processes in these populations either prior to conducting larger RCTs or to include them as potential treatment variables.

There is also a growing body of evidence demonstrating that ACT interventions may improve adherence to self-management in chronic health conditions, such as Type II diabetes[64,65] and colorectal cancer.[66,67] Gregg et al[65] conducted an RCT evaluating a single four-hour workshop combining education about diabetes self-care and acceptance and mindfulness-based skills for people with diabetes, also in a low-income community in the United States. Compared to education alone, participants in the ACT education group were more likely to use acceptance and mindfulness-based skills to respond to unwanted thoughts and feelings, reported better diabetes self-care, and showed significantly greater improvements in glycated hemoglobin (HgbA1c) control at three-months follow-up, achieving a moderate effect size. In addition, further analyses demonstrated that changes in acceptance and self-management behavior mediated the impact of treatment on changes in HgbA1c.

In another RCT, the effectiveness of a telephone-delivered coaching intervention incorporating elements of ACT that aimed to change physical activity, weight management, dietary habits, alcohol, and smoking was compared to usual care for colorectal cancer survivors.[66] The intervention consisted of 11 sessions over a period of six months. Significant effects were observed for increases in moderate physical activity and positive changes in a range of physiological dietary measures (body mass index, energy from total fat and energy from saturated fat) in the ACT intervention group at 12 months follow-up. In addition, vegetable intake significantly increased at six months. However, there were no group differences at 6 or 12 months for health-related quality of life; cancer-related fatigue; fruit, fiber, or alcohol intake; or smoking. The results of these studies are encouraging given that diabetes and colorectal cancer require the person to engage in a complex range of adherence behaviors, where medication taking, a diet and exercise program, or advice from healthcare professionals are frequently not followed as prescribed.

Within a slightly different set of applications, ACT appears promising for improved outcomes in several other public health problems that include significant adherence challenges, such as such as smoking cessation,[68–72] substance misuse,[73] and weight management.[74–76]

Smoking-cessation interventions in particular are well known for their wide-reaching implementation but low relative effectiveness. Smoking is a problem behavior that has been notoriously difficult to change in a sustained fashion—and this appears to reflect a prototype example of nonadherence. While previous studies have shown promising efficacy for face-to-face individual or group-based ACT interventions for smoking cessation,[70–72] Bricker and colleagues[71] more recently conducted a double-blind pilot RCT comparing a web-based ACT smoking cessation (Webquit. org) intervention to the National Cancer Institute's program (Smokefree. gov), which is the US national standard for web-based smoking cessation interventions.[68,69] Although participant retention was modest, findings indicated the 30-day quit rate in the ACT program was more than double that of the Smokefree.gov intervention at three months post-randomization (23% vs. 10%), and this difference was greater for those individuals who accessed the website for the recommended number of times (41% vs. 0%). Furthermore, mediation analyses showed that 80% of effects observed were accounted for by changes in acceptance of thoughts, feelings, and physical sensations. This finding is consistent with a subsequent RCT showing that an app-based version of Webquit.org (SmartQuit) was also superior to QuitGuide (Smokefree.org's app-equivalent).[69] These interventions, as with short ACT workshops for diabetes[65] and weight loss,[76] generally show medium effect sizes. This is encouraging, since the evaluated interventions are brief, easy to access, and require only very limited therapist support. If results like these continue to accumulate, ACT could prove to be potentially cost-effective for other adherence-related problems.

CONCLUSIONS

A fair summary of the adherence literature in general health contexts and in relation to chronic pain is that there are many theoretical models of adherence, many variables are implicated, and there are many intervention studies. Even so, evidence largely from systematic reviews and meta-analyses suggest that key high-utility targets for intervention are slow to emerge and current interventions are limited in their effectiveness.[4,8]

Certainly there is no such thing as a nonadherent personality[6]—perhaps that would make the problem simpler if there were. Instead, it is clear that adherence in relation to chronic pain is a highly complex process, a result of highly individualized combinations of sensory, cognitive, emotional, skills, and capacities-related, goal-related, social, cultural, socioeconomic, illness, and treatment-related factors. So far no one model has incorporated all of these in an effective fashion.

We draw a kind of implied distinction between a series of more or less conventional health behavior models, including the Theory of Planned Behavior, the Self-Regulatory Model, the Necessity Concerns Framework, and the Capability Opportunity Motivation Model on the one hand and a broader model of human performance and well-being on the other, in this case the PF Model. Each approach here has its advantages and disadvantages. None is currently dominant over the others in terms of evidence. Whether one is better than another as a guide for future work is a matter that can only be tested by applying them and observing progress made over time. We have argued elsewhere that the PF Model appears to have advantages in integrating current knowledge, feeding further study, and providing a potentially progressive approach to research strategy.[47] We point out that apparent wide-ranging benefits from applications of PF (in the form of ACT), in HIV, cancer, diabetes, weight management, physical exercise, and smoking cessation appear highly promising. Psychological flexibility includes highly integrating core processes that reduce many variables into a few core dimensions. It also has broad applicability. It is not just a model of adherence but a model that is applicable to chronic pain itself and the many collateral conditions that appear with it, including depression, anxiety, addiction, fatigue, and other chronic physical symptoms.[77] It also may have applicability to treatment staff performance and well-being.[78,79] This broad applicability is important as it creates connections between different areas of research in health and functioning, and it means that treatment providers do not need to learn and apply different models to different symptoms or behavior change challenges.

For the future, researchers may investigate and optimize factors within therapeutic interactions,[10] and perhaps the development of technological solutions, to enhance process of behavior change and persistence that interact more favorably with treatment requirements. In the end, we feel it will be innovations in theory and process that will support a leap forward, leading to improvements in how we conceptualize the problem and define key principles for treatment design. We suggest that these innovations will begin with defining adherence not as a unique and separate problem of health behavior but as fundamentally the same as any human behavioral performance problem. In each case, the problem is how to create the capacity to reinforce and maintain healthful behavior or change maladaptive behavior to meet identified goals, both in a way that is sensitive and responsive to what is present in real-time situations and not excessively restricted by our own thoughts and feelings.

REFERENCES

1. Epstein LH, Cluss PA. A behavioral medicine perspective on adherence to long-term medical regimens. *J Consult Clin Psychol.* 1982;50(6):950.
2. McDonald HP, Garg AX, Haynes RB. Interventions to enhance patient adherence to medication prescriptions: scientific review. *JAMA.* 2002;288(22):2868–2879.
3. Sabaté E. *Adherence to Long-Term Therapies: Evidence for Action.* Geneva: World Health Organization; 2003:3.
4. Broekmans S, Dobbels F, Milisen K, Morlion B, Vanderschueren S. Medication adherence in patients with chronic non-malignant pain: is there a problem? *Eur J Pain.* 2009;13(2):115–123.
5. Turk DC, Rudy TE. Neglected topics in the treatment of chronic pain patients—relapse, noncompliance, and adherence enhancement. *Pain.* 1991;44(1):5–28.
6. Unni EJ, Shiyanbola O, Farris KB. Medication adherence: a complex behavior of medication and illness beliefs. *Aging Health.* 2013;9(4):377–387.
7. Gearing RE, El-Bassel N, Ghesquiere A, Baldwin S, Gillies J, Ngeow E. Major ingredients of fidelity: a review and scientific guide to improving quality of intervention research implementation. *Clin Psychol Rev.* 2011;31(1):79–88.
8. Nieuwlaat R, Wilczynski N, Navarro T, et al. Interventions for enhancing medication adherence. *Cochrane Database Syst Rev.* 2014;11:CD000011.

9.   Zwikker HE, van den Bemt BJ, Vriezekolk JE, van den Ende CH, van Dulmen S. Psychosocial predictors of non-adherence to chronic medication: systematic review of longitudinal studies. *Patient Prefer Adherence*. 2014;8:519–563.

10. Butow P, Sharpe L. The impact of communication on adherence in pain management. *Pain*. 2013;154:S101–S107.

11. Kardas P, Lewek P, Matyjaszczyk M. Determinants of patient adherence: a review of systematic reviews. *Front Pharmacol*. 2013;4:91.

12. Petrie KJ, Perry K, Broadbent E, Weinman J. A text message programme designed to modify patients' illness and treatment beliefs improves self-reported adherence to asthma preventer medication. *Brit J Health Psych*. 2012;17(1):74–84.

13. Lehane E, McCarthy G. Intentional and unintentional medication non-adherence: a comprehensive framework for clinical research and practice? A discussion paper. *Int J Nurs Stud*. 2007;44(8):1468–1477.

14. Ajzen I. Theory of planned behavior. *Handb Theor Soc Psychol*. Vol. One. 2011;1:438.

15. Leventhal H, Nerenz DR, Steele DJ. *Illness Representations and Coping with Health Threats*. Hillsdale, NJ: Erlbaum; 1984.

16. Molloy GJ, Messerli-Bürgy N, Hutton G, Wikman A, Perkins-Porras L, Steptoe A. Intentional and unintentional non-adherence to medications following an acute coronary syndrome: a longitudinal study. *J. Psychosom Res*. 2014;76(5):430–432.

17. Schroeder K, Fahey T, Ebrahim S. Interventions for improving adherence to treatment in patients with high blood pressure in ambulatory settings. *Cochrane Database Syst Rev*. 2004;2:CD004804.

18. Petrie KJ, Weinman J. Patients' perceptions of their illness: the dynamo of volition in health care. *Curr Dir Psychol Sci*. February 1, 2012;21(1):60–65.

19. Cecil DW. Relational control patterns in physician–patient clinical encounters: continuing the conversation. *Health Commun*. 1998;10(2):125–149.

20. Monane M, Bohn RL, Gurwitz JH, Glynn RJ, Levin R, Avorn J. Compliance with antihypertensive therapy among elderly Medicaid enrollees: the roles of age, gender, and race. *Am J Public Health*. 1996;86(12):1805–1808.

21. Svensson S, Kjellgren KI, Ahlner J, Säljö R. Reasons for adherence with antihypertensive medication. *Int J Cardiol*. 2000;76(2):157–163.

22. Rich A, Brandes K, Mullan B, Hagger MS. Theory of planned behavior and adherence in chronic illness: a meta-analysis. *J Behav Med*. 2015;38(4):673–688.

23. Gonzalez JS, Batchelder AW, Psaros C, Safren SA. Depression and HIV/AIDS treatment nonadherence: a review and meta-analysis. *J ACQ Immun Def Synd*. 2011;58(2).

24. Rogers RE. *The Theory of Planned Behavior and Adherence to a Multidisciplinary Treatment Program for Chronic Pain* [master's thesis]. Denton: Univeristy of North Texas; 2005. http://digital.library.unt.edu/ark:/67531/metadc4936/m1/49/.

25. Brandes K, Mullan B. Can the common-sense model predict adherence in chronically ill patients? A meta-analysis. *Health Psychol Rev*. 2014;8(2):129–153.

26. Graham CD, Simmons Z, Stuart SR, Rose MR. The potential of psychological interventions to improve quality of life and mood in muscle disorders. *Muscle Nerve*. 2015;52(1):131–136.

27. Horne R, Cooper V, Gellaitry G, Date HL, Fisher M. Patients' perceptions of highly active antiretroviral therapy in relation to treatment uptake and adherence: the utility of the necessity-concerns framework. *J ACQ Immun Def Synd*. 2007;45(3):334–341.

28. Horne R, Weinman J. Patients' beliefs about prescribed medicines and their role in adherence to treatment in chronic physical illness. *J Psychosom. Res.* 1999;47(6):555–567.

29. Horne R, Weinman J, Hankins M. The beliefs about medicines questionnaire: the development and evaluation of a new method for assessing the cognitive representation of medication. *Psychol Health.* 1999;14(1):1–24.

30. Horne R, Chapman SC, Parham R, Freemantle N, Forbes A, Cooper V. Understanding patients' adherence-related beliefs about medicines prescribed for long-term conditions: a meta-analytic review of the Necessity-Concerns Framework. *PLoS One.* 2013;8(12):e80633.

31. Easthall C, Song F, Bhattacharya D. A meta-analysis of cognitive-based behaviour change techniques as interventions to improve medication adherence. *BMJ Open.* 2013;3(8):e002749.

32. Brown I, Sheeran P, Reuber M. Enhancing antiepileptic drug adherence: a randomized controlled trial. *Epilepsy Behav.* 2009;16(4):634–639.

33. Bisonó AM, Manuel JK, Forcehimes AA, O'Donohue W, Levensky E. Promoting treatment adherence through motivational interviewing. In: O'Donohue, Levensky, E, eds. *Promoting Treatment Adherence: A Practical Handbook for Health Care Providers.* Thousand Oaks, CA: SAGE; 2006:71–84.

34. Michie S, van Stralen MM, West R. The behaviour change wheel: a new method for characterising and designing behaviour change interventions. *Implement Sci.* 2011;6(1):42.

35. Jackson C, Eliasson L, Barber N, Weinman J. Applying COM-B to medication adherence: a suggested framework for research and interventions. *Eur Health Psychol.* 2014;16(1):7–17.

36. McCracken LM, Hoskins J, Eccleston C. Concerns about medication and medication use in chronic pain. *J Pain.* 2006;7(10):726–734.

37. Rosser BA, McCracken LM, Velleman SC, Boichat C, Eccleston C. Concerns about medication and medication adherence in patients with chronic pain recruited from general practice. *Pain.* 2011;152(5):1201–1205.

38. Broekmans S, Dobbels F, Milisen K, Morlion B, Vanderschueren S. Pharmacologic pain treatment in a multidisciplinary pain center: do patients adhere to the prescription of the physician? *Clin J Pain.* 2010;26(2):81–86.

39. Spoelstra SL, Schueller M, Hilton M, Ridenour K. Interventions combining motivational interviewing and cognitive behaviour to promote medication adherence: a literature review. *J Clin Nurs.* 2015;24(9–10):1163–1173.

40. Curran C, Williams AC, Potts HW. Cognitive-behavioral therapy for persistent pain: does adherence after treatment affect outcome? *Eur J Pain.* 2009;13(2):178–188.

41. Nicholas MK, Asghari A, Corbett M, et al. Is adherence to pain self-management strategies associated with improved pain, depression and disability in those with disabling chronic pain? *Eur J Pain.* 2012;16(1):93–104.

42. Kerns RD, Burns JW, Shulman M, et al. Can we improve cognitive-behavioral therapy for chronic back pain treatment engagement and adherence? A controlled trial of tailored versus standard therapy. *Health Psychol.* 2014;33(9):938.

43. Hayes SC, Strosahl, K, Wilson, KG. *Acceptance and Commitment Therapy: An Experiential Approach to Behavior Change.* New York: Guilford; 1999.

44. Hayes SC, Luoma JB, Bond FW, Masuda A, Lillis J. Acceptance and Commitment Therapy: model, processes and outcomes. *Behav Res Ther.* 2006;44(1):1–25.

45. McCracken LM. Learning to live with pain: acceptance of pain predicts adjustment in persons with chronic pain. *Pain.* 1998;74(1):21–27.

46. Hann KE, McCracken LM. A systematic review of randomized controlled trials of Acceptance and Commitment Therapy for adults with chronic pain: outcome domains, design quality, and efficacy. *J Contextual Behav Sci.* 2014;3(4):217–227.

47. McCracken LM, Morley S. The Psychological Flexibility Model: a basis for integration and progress in psychological approaches to chronic pain management. *J Pain.* 2014;15(3):221–234.

48. Öst L-G. The efficacy of Acceptance and Commitment Therapy: an updated systematic review and meta-analysis. *Behav Res Ther.* 2014;61:105–121.

49. Davis M, Morina N, Powers M, Smits J, Emmelkamp P. A meta-analysis of the efficacy of Acceptance and Commitment Therapy for clinically relevant mental and physical health problems. *Psychother Psychosom.* 2015;84(1):30–36.

50. Powers MB, Zum Vörde Sive Vörding MB, Emmelkamp PM. Acceptance and commitment therapy: a meta-analytic review. *Psychother Psychosom.* 2009;78(2):73–80.

51. Prevedini AB, Presti G, Rabitti E, Miselli G, Moderato P. Acceptance and Commitment Therapy (ACT): the foundation of the therapeutic model and an overview of its contribution to the treatment of patients with chronic physical diseases. *G Ital Med Lav Ergon.* 2011;33(1 Suppl A):A53–A63.

52. Hayes SC, Barnes-Holmes D, Roche B. *Relational Frame Theory: A Post-Skinnerian Account of Human Language and Cognition.* London: Kluwer; 2001.

53. Hayes SC. *Analytic Goals and the Varieties of Scientific Contextualism.* Reno, NV: Context Press; 1993.

54. Hayes SC, Levin ME, Plumb-Vilardaga J, Villatte JL, Pistorello J. Acceptance and Commitment Therapy and contextual behavioral science: examining the progress of a distinctive model of behavioral and cognitive therapy. *Behav Ther.* 2013;44(2):180–198.

55. Scott W, McCracken LM. Psychological flexibility, Acceptance and Commitment Therapy, and chronic pain. *Curr Opin Psychol.* 2015;2:91–96.

56. McCracken LM. *Acceptance and Commitment Therapy and Mindfulness: Specific Processes, Evidence, and Methods*: Hoboken, NJ: Wiley; 2014.

57. McCracken LM. *Mindfulness and Acceptance in Behavioral Medicine: Current Theory and Practice.* Oakland, CA: New Harbinger; 2011.

58. McCracken LM. Committed action: an application of the Psychological Flexibility Model to activity patterns in chronic pain. *J Pain.* 2013;14(8), 828–835.

59. Hayes SC, Villatte M, Levin M, Hildebrandt M. Open, aware, and active: contextual approaches as an emerging trend in the behavioral and cognitive therapies. *Annu Rev Clin Psychol.* 2011;7:141–168.

60. Scott W, McCracken LM, Norton S. A confirmatory factor analysis of facets of psychological flexibility in a sample of people seeking treatment for chronic pain. *Ann Behav Med.* 2015:1–12.

61. Gillanders D. Acceptance and Commitment Therapy and motivational interviewing for mindfulness and acceptance in behavioral medicine. *Curr Theory Practice.* 2011:217.

62. Nelson C, Kenowitz J, Mulhall J. Acceptance and Commitment Therapy (ACT) for adherence to an erectile rehabilitation program (ERP) after radical

prostatectomy (RP) (paper presented at the annual meeting of the Scientific Meeting of the Sexual Medicine Society of North America), Nov. 2014.

63. Moitra E, Herbert JD, Forman EM. Acceptance-based behavior therapy to promote HIV medication adherence. *AIDS Care.* 2011;23(12):1660–1667.

64. Nes AA, van Dulmen S, Eide E, et al. The development and feasibility of a web-based intervention with diaries and situational feedback via smartphone to support self-management in patients with diabetes type 2. *Diabetes Res Clin Pract.* 2012;97(3):385–393.

65. Gregg JA, Callaghan GM, Hayes SC, Glenn-Lawson JL. Improving diabetes self-management through acceptance, mindfulness, and values: a randomized controlled trial. *J Consult Clin Psychol.* 2007;75(2):336.

66. Hawkes AL, Chambers SK, Pakenham KI, et al. Effects of a telephone-delivered multiple health behavior change intervention (CanChange) on health and behavioral outcomes in survivors of colorectal cancer: a randomized controlled trial. *J Clin Oncol.* 2013;31(18):2313–2321.

67. Hawkes AL, Pakenham KI, Chambers SK, Patrao TA, Courneya KS. Effects of a multiple health behavior change intervention for colorectal cancer survivors on psychosocial outcomes and quality of life: a randomized controlled trial. *Ann Behav Med.* 2014;48(3):359–370.

68. Bricker J, Wyszynski C, Comstock B, Heffner JL. Pilot randomized controlled trial of web-based Acceptance and Commitment Therapy for smoking cessation. *Nicotine Tob Res.* 2013;15(10):1756–1764.

69. Bricker JB, Mull KE, Kientz JA, et al. Randomized, controlled pilot trial of a smartphone app for smoking cessation using Acceptance and Commitment Therapy. *Drug Alcohol Depend.* 2014;143:87–94.

70. Gifford EV, Kohlenberg BS, Hayes SC, et al. Acceptance-based treatment for smoking cessation. *Behav Ther.* 2004;35(4):689–705.

71. Bricker JB, Mann SL, Marek PM, Liu J, Peterson AV. Telephone-delivered Acceptance and Commitment Therapy for adult smoking cessation: a feasibility study. *Nicotine Tob Res.* 2010;12(4):454–458.

72. Hernández-López M, Luciano MC, Bricker JB, Roales-Nieto JG, Montesinos F. Acceptance and Commitment Therapy for smoking cessation: a preliminary study of its effectiveness in comparison with cognitive behavioral therapy. *Psychol Addict Behav.* 2009;23(4):723.

73. Hayes SC, Wilson KG, Gifford EV, et al. A preliminary trial of twelve-step facilitation and Acceptance and Commitment Therapy with polysubstance-abusing methadone-maintained opiate addicts. *Behav Ther.* 2004;35(4):667–688.

74. Forman EM, Butryn ML, Hoffman KL, Herbert JD. An open trial of an acceptance-based behavioral intervention for weight loss. *Cogn Behav Pract.* 2009;16(2):223–235.

75. Forman E, Butryn M, Juarascio A, et al. The mind your health project: a randomized controlled trial of an innovative behavioral treatment for obesity. *Obesity.* 2013;21(6):1119–1126.

76. Lillis J, Hayes SC, Bunting K, Masuda A. Teaching acceptance and mindfulness to improve the lives of the obese: a preliminary test of a theoretical model. *Ann Behav Med.* 2009;37(1):58–69.

77. Hayes SC, Pistorello J, Levin ME. Acceptance and Commitment Therapy as a unified model of behavior change. *Couns Psychol.* 2012;40(7):976–1002.

78. McCracken LM, Yang S-Y. A contextual cognitive-behavioral analysis of rehabilitation workers' health and well-being: influences of acceptance, mindfulness, and values-based action. *Rehabil Psychol.* 2008;53(4):479.

79. Barker E, McCracken LM. From traditional cognitive–behavioural therapy to Acceptance and Commitment Therapy for chronic pain: a mixed-methods study of staff experiences of change. *Brit J Pain.* 2013:2049463713498865.

CHAPTER 3

✿

Adherence in Pharmacotherapy

Maximizing Benefit and Minimizing Risk

MARC O. MARTEL AND ROBERT N. JAMISON

INTRODUCTION

Over the past few decades, pharmacotherapy has become the cornerstone of chronic pain management. Adherence to pharmacotherapy, however, is pivotal in order to optimize pain management outcomes and minimize any potential risks associated with medication use. In this chapter, we begin with a brief definition of key terms relevant for a discussion on pharmacotherapy adherence. The factors associated an increased risk for adherence problems among patients with pain are then discussed, and an overview of screening instruments and strategies that can be used for the assessment and management of patients at risk of medication nonadherence is presented. Given that research on pharmacotherapy adherence among patients with pain has predominantly been conducted in the context of opioid therapy, a particular emphasis is placed on opioids. However, issues associated with adherence to nonopioid pharmacotherapies are also addressed throughout the various sections of this chapter.

DEFINITIONS

Pharmacotherapy Adherence

Treatment adherence broadly refers to an active, voluntary, collaborative involvement of the patient in a mutually acceptable course of behavior to produce a desired preventative or therapeutic result. In the context of pharmacotherapy, treatment adherence (i.e., medication adherence) refers to the use of medications as prescribed or directed.

Aberrant Drug Behaviors

Aberrant drug behaviors refer to a wide range of erratic behaviors exhibited by patients in relation to their prescribed medications. Some of these behaviors may include requesting early refills, losing prescriptions, or seeking prescription drugs from multiple physicians. Although aberrant drug behaviors may be simply due to error or misunderstanding, they may also be due to more serious problems such as drug misuse, drug addiction, or diversion.

Prescription Drug Misuse

Prescription drug misuse refers to the use of prescription drugs in a manner other than how they are indicated or prescribed. Prescription drug misuse, also sometimes termed "nonadherence," includes behaviors such as taking higher doses of medications than prescribed, using medications for symptoms other than pain (e.g., to improve mood or sleep), and using unsanctioned substances in addition to the prescribed medication regimen.

Prescription Drug Abuse

Prescription drug abuse refers to the use of prescription drugs, without the supervision of a physician, for recreational or nonmedical purposes. A typical example would be an individual who occasionally takes prescription opioids provided by friends or family members solely to experience the potentially pleasurable or euphoric effects of opioids.

Prescription Drug Addiction

Addiction has been defined by the Liaison Committee in Pain and Addiction conjointly formed by the American Pain Society, American Academy of Pain Medicine, and the American Society of Addiction Medicine as a chronic neurobiological disease with genetic, psychosocial, and environmental factors influencing its development and manifestations. It is characterized by behaviors that include one or more of the following: impaired control over drug use, compulsive use, continued use despite harm, and craving. From a diagnostic standpoint, addiction refers to patients meeting criteria for a diagnosis of substance use disorder based on the nosological system put forward by the American Psychiatric Association in the *Diagnostic and Statistical Manual of Mental Disorders* (DSM). For instance, patients prescribed opioids or benzodiazepines who exhibit aberrant drug behaviors may (or not) meet criteria for an opioid use disorder or a sedative-hypnotic use disorder, respectively.

OVERVIEW OF FACTORS ASSOCIATED WITH MEDICATION NONADHERENCE

Opioid Medications

Opioid analgesics refer to a broad class of drugs including (a) alkaloids extracted from poppy seeds (morphine, codeine) and their semisynthetic derivatives (oxycodone, hydromorphone, oxymorphone) and (b) synthetic phenlypiperidines (meperidine, fentanyl) and synthetic pseudopiperidines such as methadone. Opioid analgesics act on three major classes of receptors: μ, δ, and κ receptors. Each of these classes of receptors has its representative endogenous ligand (e.g., endorphin for the μ receptor and dynorphin for the κ receptor). These classes of opioid receptors are widely distributed throughout the central and peripheral nervous system as well as other systems such as the gastrointestinal tract. Based on their pharmacodynamic profiles, opioid analgesics can also be classified as a full agonist at opioid receptors (e.g., morphine, fentanyl) or an agonist-antagonist such as buprenorphine.

The use of opioids for the management of chronic noncancer pain has increased exponentially over the past few decades in North America. Despite the potential benefits of opioids, the rise in the use of opioids has been accompanied by escalating rates of prescription opioid misuse and addiction among patients with chronic pain. Opioid misuse and addiction may lead to numerous adverse consequences, including serious health problems, and may ultimately result in opioid-related overdose death. Rates of opioid misuse and addiction among patients with pain treated with opioids have long been assumed to be negligible due to a number of widely cited case reports and observational studies published during the 1980s in which these problems were claimed to be very low or even inexistent. Over the past few years, however, many authors have expressed skepticism toward these low estimates, and it is now widely acknowledged that early estimates of misuse and addiction were far too low. As pointed out by Sullivan,[61] one of the reasons these estimates were too low is because they were derived from unrepresentative populations of chronic pain patients treated with opioids. For instance, early estimates of opioid misuse or addiction were based on studies that excluded "high-risk" patients, such as those with mental health issues or past history of substance use problems. Given that these patients are particularly likely to be prescribed opioids in real-life clinical scenarios, it is reasonable to argue that early studies yielded artificially low estimates of prescription opioid misuse and addiction.

To date, there are very few large-scale studies that have been conducted to reliably determine rates of addiction among patients with pain. While rates of aberrant drug behaviors and opioid misuse have been found to be up to 40 % to 60% in primary and tertiary care settings,[64] much less is known on rates of opioid addiction. In a recently published systematic review of the literature, Vowles et al.[67] found a wide variability in prescription opioid addiction rates across studies (i.e., range: 8 % to 34.1%). The differences observed in opioid addiction rates across studies are assumed to be due, in part, to differences in study populations, study designs, and settings in which opioids were prescribed. While uncertainty remains about the true rates of opioid addiction among patients with pain, early misuse of opioids may in some cases subsequently lead to opioid addiction, supporting the need for early risk assessment, very careful monitoring, and strategies in place to assess and improve compliance when indicated.

Risk Factors for Prescription Opioid Misuse and Addiction

In the literature and the media, it is often implied that problems such as opioid misuse and addiction are directly caused by the "addictive potential" of opioids. Although the basic pharmacokinetic properties of opioid analgesics are known to be associated with an increased potential for misuse and/or addiction, many patients prescribed high doses of opioids do not exhibit problematic opioid use behaviors. It is pivotal to understand that the determinants of opioid misuse and addiction rest with the user and that many patient-specific factors may increase susceptibility to these problems. The following is an overview of the demographic and psychologic factors known to be associated with an increased risk for opioid misuse and addiction among patients with chronic pain prescribed opioids.

Demographic and background factors

Research has revealed that chronic pain patients at increased risk for opioid misuse and/or addiction include those who are (a) younger (b) single, (c) less educated, (d) unemployed and those with (e) a personal or family history of substance use problems, such as smoking, heavy drinking, or illicit drug use. Patients with a history of (f) sexual or physical abuse (g) criminal or legal problems, (h) risk-taking or thrill-seeking behaviors, and (i) who are in frequent contact with high-risk individuals or environments are also at increased risk for opioid misuse and addiction.[7,35,36,64]

Psychological disturbances

Studies conducted among chronic pain patients indicate that up to 65% of patients meet diagnostic criteria for one (or more) comorbid psychiatric disorder, with mood disorders, anxiety disorders, and personality disorders being among the most prevalent.[22] While a few recent studies have found that personality disorders are associated with an increased risk for prescription opioid misuse,[63,75] the most consistent finding that has emerged from previous studies among patients with pain is the association between anxiety and depressive symptoms (i.e., negative affect) and prescription opioid misuse. Findings from several studies have indicated that patients with high levels of negative affect are two to three times more likely to misuse prescription opioids than patients with low levels of negative affect.[25,69,74] Symptoms of negative affect have also been found to be associated with an increased likelihood of meeting criteria for an opioid use disorder.[6,26] Among patients with pain, other psychological factors have also been found to be associated with an increased risk for prescription opioid misuse and/or addiction, including catastrophizing[50] and somatization.[48]

Preexisting personality traits

There is reason to believe that patients with high negative affect hold pre-existing personality traits that make them prone to misusing opioids or to become addicted to their opioid medication. For example, some studies have found that individuals with high negative affect are characterized by heightened impulsivity and sensation-seeking, two personality traits that have consistently been identified as risk factors for various types of substance use problems.[65]

Opioid craving

Findings from recent studies suggest that opioid craving might also be responsible, in part, for the association between negative affect and problematic opioid use. The concept of craving, which refers to the subjective desire to consume certain substances, has long been invoked in the substance use literature to explain the development and persistence of problems such as alcoholism, smoking, and illicit drug use (for a review, see Drummond[23] and Tiffany and Wray[62]). Among patients with chronic pain prescribed long-term opioid therapy, negative affect has been associated with heightened reports of opioid craving,[49,71] and craving has been associated with various indices of misuse, including patient reports of opioid misuse,[49,70,71] physician ratings of opioid misuse behaviors,[71] and abnormal urine toxicology screens.[12,70,71] In a recent study,[49] opioid craving was found to mediate the association between negative affect and opioid misuse, which suggests that craving might contribute to the increased rates of prescription opioid misuse observed among patients with high levels of negative affect.

Nonopioid Medications

In addition to opioids, the pharmacological management of chronic pain patients may also include several other analgesic and nonanalgesic medications, such as sedatives-hypnotics, antidepressants, anticonvulsants, muscle relaxants, and nonsteroidal anti-inflammatory drugs (NSAIDs). To date, research on pharmacotherapy adherence among patients with pain has predominantly been conducted in the context of opioid therapy, but a few studies have examined adherence-related issues among patients with chronic pain prescribed sedative-hypnotic drugs such as benzodiazepines or barbiturates. Some studies have also examined adherence-related issues among headache pain patients prescribed headache medications such as ergotamine and triptans. To our knowledge, very few studies have examined pharmacotherapy adherence to NSAIDs, antidepressants, or anticonvulsants among patients with pain. As a result, evidence is insufficient to draw reliable and meaningful conclusions with regard to adherence issues in the context of these pharmacological treatments. The following sections thus solely focus on adherence issues associated with the prescription of sedatives-hypnotics (i.e., benzodiazepines, barbiturates) and headache medications (e.g., ergotamine, triptans) among patients with pain.

Sedative-Hypnotics

Sedative-hypnotics such as benzodiazepines and barbiturates are centrally acting drugs that act through modulation of the $GABA_A$ receptor to enhance the activity of GABA, an inhibitory neurotransmitter involved in the experience of sedative and hypnotic effects. Benzodiazepines, which have progressively been replacing barbiturates, provide only weak analgesic benefits but are commonly used to treat anxiety and insomnia both among patients with pain and without pain conditions.[32,52] Large-scale survey data indicate that roughly 40% of patients with pain on long-term opioid therapy are concurrently prescribed benzodiazepines,[24,28,56] in part due to the high prevalence of anxiety- and sleep-related problems in this population. When benzodiazepines are used in combination with opioids, they may contribute to enhancing the subjective effects of opioids, such as "drug liking" and "euphoria."[32,40,47] The co-prescribing of opioids and benzodiazepines may be indicated in some cases but may be accompanied by significant risks when these drugs are either misused (e.g., overused) or ingested in combination with unsanctioned substances. For instance, evidence indicates that opioid-related deaths most commonly involve co-ingestion of additional substances such as sedatives, alcohol, or illicit drugs,[13,72,73] with the most lethal combination of polysubstance overdose being the combined use of opioids and benzodiazepines.[13]

A few studies have been conducted in order to examine the prevalence of problematic sedative-hypnotic use among patients with chronic pain. For instance, Kouyanou et al.[43] conducted one of the first studies in this area and found that 12% of chronic pain patients either misused their benzodiazepines or met DSM (third edition) criteria for benzodiazepine abuse and/or dependence. A similar prevalence rate was recently observed by Nielsen et al.,[52] with 10% of chronic pain patients reporting having at least once used their benzodiazepines differently from how they were prescribed.

In the latter study, 9% of daily benzodiazepine users were found to meet diagnostic criteria for a lifetime benzodiazepine use disorder using the International Classification of Diseases (ICD) criteria. These data are consistent with those of Liebschutz et al.,[46] who found that 11% of chronic pain patients treated in primary care settings meet DSM (fourth edition; DSM-IV) criteria for a sedative-use disorder involving either benzodiazepines or barbiturates.

To date, little research has been conducted on the risk factors for problematic sedative-hypnotic use among patients with chronic pain. Studies have been conducted on the factors associated with the co-prescribing of sedative-hypnotic drugs (e.g., benzodiazepines) and opioids in patients with pain,[24,28,56] but these studies did not assess problematic drug use outcomes. In one of the few studies conducted in this area, depressive symptoms have been found to be associated with elevated rates of prescription drug misuse and prescription drug use disorders,[43] but these problematic prescription drug use outcomes were not specific to sedative-hypnotic drugs. In another study, Liebschutz et al.[46] found that chronic pain patients meeting criteria for a prescription drug use disorder were more likely to be young, to have a personal or family history of substance use problems, to smoke cigarettes, to have served jail time, and to have mental health issues. Once again, though, the diagnosis of prescription drug use disorder was not limited to sedative-hypnotic drug use, as it also included problematic opioid use. It thus remains uncertain whether the patient-specific factors noted here are specifically associated with an increased risk for a sedative-hypnotic use disorder, with the likelihood of meeting criteria for an opioid use disorder, or both. Additional research will be needed in order to further elucidate the factors specifically associated with problematic sedative-hypnotic use among patients with chronic pain.

Headache Medications

Medications such as ergotamine and triptans are frequently prescribed for patients experiencing headaches. There has been several reports of headache patients overusing ergotamine and triptan medications, leading to a condition termed medication overuse headaches (MOH) in roughly 40% to 50% of patients seen in specialized headache centers and outpatient neurology clinics. MOH is a condition characterized by an increase in headache frequency and severity, which may lead to significant distress and disability. The diagnosis of MOH is typically made based on the International Classification of Headache Disorders criteria proposed by the International Headache Society. To date, very little research has been conducted on the factors associated with MOH among patients overusing ergotamine and triptan medications. The few studies conducted in this area have revealed that the likelihood of MOH is greater among women,[16,20] among patients with more severe headache and/or migraine pains,[55] and among patients with sleeping problems,[60] poor coping skills,[44] and mental health issues.[18,54]

SCREENING FOR PATIENTS AT RISK OF MEDICATION NONADHERENCE BEFORE INITIATING PHARMACOTHERAPY

As noted earlier, the determinants of medication nonadherence rest with the user, and many patient-specific factors may increase susceptibility to these problems. A number of instruments have been developed to assess risks of medication nonadherence and/or problematic prescription drug use behaviors before initiating pharmacotherapy. The vast majority of these instruments, however, have been specifically developed and validated for patients prescribed long-term opioid therapy. As discussed next, instruments are available to assess adherence issues in the context of other pharmacological treatments (e.g., sedative-hypnotics), but these instruments are not considered "screening tools" as they are generally used after the initiation of treatment.

Opioid-Specific Instruments

Many physicians struggle with providing appropriate pain relief for patients while minimizing the misuse of opioid analgesics, and, in response, concerted efforts have been made to identify those individuals at risk for problematic opioid use behaviors. A number of regulatory and professional organizations have released recommendations and guidelines related to the use of opioids among patients with chronic pain.[14,29] These guidelines emphasize the importance of opioid risk assessment before initiation of long-term opioid therapy. In addition to performing a thorough medical history, a review of past medical records, and a medical examination, an opioid risk assessment using validated screening tools is recommended. Some of the most commonly used tools include the Screener and Opioid Assessment for Patients with Pain—Revised (SOAPP-R)[12]; the Opioid Risk Tool (ORT)[74]; the Diagnosis, Intractability, Risk, and Efficacy (DIRE) scale[3]; and the Screening Instrument for Substance Abuse Potential (SISAP).[15] Scores on any of these instruments are not necessarily a reason to deny opioids but instead allow clinicians to identify patients who might need close monitoring in order to minimize the likelihood of opioid misuse or addiction. More detailed information on each of these instruments is provided in the following sections as well as in Table 3.1.

The SOAPP-R[12] is a self-administered 24-item screening tool developed and validated for those persons with chronic pain who are being considered

Table 3.1. SCREENING TOOLS FOR IDENTIFYING PATIENTS AT RISK OF PRESCRIPTION OPIOID MISUSE OR ADDICTION

Name	Description	Scoring
Screener and Opioid Assessment for Patients with Pain—Revised[20]	• Completed by the patient • 24-item questionnaire • Items designed to capture eight domains, including substance abuse history, psychiatric history, crimimal history, medication-related behaviors, doctor–patient relationship, emotional attachment to pain medications, personal care and lifestyle issues, and psychosocial problems	• Any individual who scores 18 or more on the this scale is considered to be at risk for opioid misuse
Opioid Risk Tool[11]	• Completed by the clinician • Five-item questionnaire • Items designed to capture patients' background characteristics and psychiatric history	• Scores suggesting risk for misuse or addiction: 0–3 = low risk 4–7 = moderate risk ≥ 8 = high risk
Diagnosis, Intractability, Risk, and Efficacy[26]	• Completed by the clinician • Seven-item checklist designed to predict future opioid-related outcomes and compliance during opioid therapy • Items capture four domains: diagnosis, intractability, efficacy, and risk. four subdomains of risk are assessed (psychological, chemical, reliability, social support).	• Scores: ≤ 13 = unsuitable candidate for opioid therapy ≥ 14 = good candidate for opioid therapy
Screening Instrument for Substance Abuse Potential[27]	• Completed by the clinician • Five-item telephone interview • Items designed to capture patients' substance abuse history	• A positive answer to any of the questions suggests risk for opioid misuse and need for further assessment

Note: Recent opioid treatment guidelines jointly released by the American Pain Society and American Academy of Pain Medicine identify all of these tools as having good content, construct, and face validity.[24]

for long-term opioid therapy. The SOAPP-R was designed to predict aberrant medication-related behaviors. This questionnaire includes subtle items that encourage the patient to admit to certain behaviors that are positively correlated with opioid misuse yet are not perceived to lead to reprisals. Any individual who scores 18 or more on the SOAPP-R is rated as being at risk for opioid misuse. This screening tool has been found to identify over 90% of those who will eventually misuse opioids. It has been cross-validated in more than 600 patients across the United States.[10] The reliability and predictive validity of the SOAPP-R, as measured by the area under the curve (AUC), were found to be highly significant (test–retest reliability = .91; coefficient α = .86; AUC = .74). These results were also sufficiently similar to values found with the initial sample (coefficient α = 88; AUC = .81). A cut-off score of 18 revealed a sensitivity of .81 and specificity of .68. Results of a cross-validation suggest that the psychometric parameters of the SOAPP-R are not based solely on the unique characteristics of the initial validation sample. In this multicenter validation study,[10] longitudinal data were collected over five months, and SOAPP-R scores were studied as prospective predictors of scores on the Aberrant Drug Behavior Index, which combines the results of a patient self-report measure of medication use, a multi-item behavioral rating scale completed by the treating physician (e.g., items include unsanctioned dose increases, multiple lost/ stolen prescriptions, etc.), and a urine toxicology screen.

The five-item ORT,[74] a brief checklist completed by the clinician, is a validated questionnaire that predicts which patients will display aberrant drug-related behaviors and/or opioid misuse behaviors over the course of opioid therapy. Scores of 8 or higher suggest high risk for opioid misuse. The DIRE[3] is a similar clinician-rating tool used to predict suitability for long-term opioid treatment for noncancer pain. Scores of 14 and higher on the DIRE suggest a greater suitability of opioid therapy for patients with pain. The SISAP[15] is also a self-report questionnaire designed to screen for substance abuse potential. A positive answer to any of the SISAP question suggests risk for opioid misuse and need for further assessment.

MONITORING MEDICATION ADHERENCE OVER THE COURSE OF TREATMENT

After conducting the initial "risk assessment," monitoring medication adherence over the course of treatment is important in order to prevent or reduce prescription drug misuse behaviors. Monitoring medication adherence may also minimize the development of more severe problems such as prescription drug addiction. A number of instruments have been developed to assess adherence problems occurring over the course of opioid and nonopioid pharmacotherapies. These instruments are described in the following sections.

The Current Opioid Misuse Measure (COMM)[11] is a questionnaire developed and validated for patients who have already been prescribed opioids for chronic pain. The 17-item COMM helps to identify those patients who are currently misusing their prescription opioids. The COMM, different from measures that were created to predict misuse behaviors in patients, is able to repeatedly document opioid compliance and to demonstrate appropriateness of opioid therapy. The COMM is a brief but useful self-report measure of current aberrant drug-related behavior. A score of 9 is used as a cutoff to identify someone at risk for current opioid misuse with a sensitivity of .76 and specificity of .66. Based on cross validation,[9] the reliability and predictive validity, as measured by the AUC, were found to be highly significant (AUC = .79) and similar to the AUC obtained in the original validation study (AUC = .81). Also, the reliability (coefficient α) was .83, which is comparable to the .86 obtained in the original study. The results of a cross-validation suggest that the psychometric parameters of the COMM are not based on the unique characteristics of the initial validation sample. A benefit of both the SOAPP-R and COMM is that they include subtle items that are correlated with opioid misuse and are items patients are willing to honestly complete.

The Opioid Compliance Checklist (OCC)[37] was devised to be a brief, self-report measure to help document opioid compliance for use by prescribing practitioners. It was initially designed to reflect the consensus of the literature as to those components of an opioid therapy agreement that would outline patients' responsibilities and clinic policies in prescribing opioids for chronic pain. The items were worded to reflect a yes/no response over the past month for aberrant drug-related behavior associated with the use of prescription opioids. The original items of the OCC were administered to 157 chronic non-cancer pain patients who were taking long-term opioids, and these patients were followed for a year to evaluate evidence of noncompliance and aberrant medication-related behavior. Among the original 157 subjects, 70 (44.6%) had a positive drug misuse index based on a positive urine toxicology results, self-report measures, and physician-rated aberrant drug-related behavior. As in previous studies,[39,71] this triangulation of data allowed for identification of patients by combining objective indicators with self-report measures to maximize the chances of accurately determining opioid misuse.

Other instruments can also be used to monitor and assess opioid misuse behaviors over the course of opioid therapy, such as the Pain Medication Questionnaire (PMQ),[1] the Prescription Drug Use Questionnaire–patient

Table 3.2. TOOLS FOR IDENTIFYING PATIENTS WHO ARE MISUSING OPIOIDS OVER THE COURSE OF THERAPY

Name	Description	Scoring
Current Opioid Misuse Measure[28]	• Completed by the patient • 17-item questionnaire designed to assess various types of opioid misuse and aberrant drug behaviors	• A score of ≥ 9 is used as a cutoff suggesting potential opioid misuse or aberrant drug behaviors
Pain Medication Questionnaire[29]	• Completed by the patient • 26 items designed to assess various types of opioid misuse and aberrant drug behaviors	• Higher scores suggest greater likelihood of opioid misuse and/or aberrant drug behaviors
Prescription Drug Use Questionnaire– Patient version[30]	• Completed by the patient • 31-item questionnaire designed to assess behaviors indicative of opioid abuse or dependence.	• A score > 10 suggests potential opioid use disorder (i.e., abuse or dependence).
Pain Assessment and Documentation Tool[31]	• Completed by the clinician • 41-item checklist designed to assess/ monitor opioid-related outcomes and compliance over the course of therapy	• No cutoff score; this scale is used for documentation purposes only
Addiction Behavior Checklist[32]	• Completed by the clinician • 20-item checklist designed to assess various types of opioid misuse and aberrant drug behaviors	• A score of ≥ 3 suggests ongoing problematic opioid use
Opioid Compliance Checklist[33]	• Completed by the patient • Five-item questionnaire to assess opioid compliance	• A positive answer to any of the items suggests ongoing opioid misuse

version (PDUQ-p),[17] the Pain Assessment and Documentation Tool (PADT),[53] and the Addiction Behavior Checklist (ABC).[76] While the PMQ and PDUQ-p can be self-administered, the PADT and ABC are questionnaires/checklists that must be completed by clinicians. More detailed information on each of these instruments in provided in Table 3.2.

Other Opioid-Related Instruments and Assessment Procedures

Urine Toxicology Screens

Urine toxicology screens are particularly useful for determining a patient's adherence to prescribed opioid medications. Immunoassay urine screens can be helpful in determining a particular class of drug present in the urine, but gas chromatology/mass spectrometry (GC/MS) is the most sensitive and specific type of urine screens and is particularly helpful in quantifying particular prescription medication. GC/MS screens are also helpful in determining creatinine levels used to identify possible drug tampering/adulteration as well as presence of illegal substances and/or absence of prescribed medications. Objectively documenting compliance by obtaining a urine screen on every patient on opioid therapy at least yearly is recommended.[14]

Random urine toxicology screening among chronic pain patients prescribed opioids has revealed a high incidence of abnormal results. In a study among 470 patients, 45% of the sample were found to have an abnormal result.[51] Another study found 21% of the study patients to have evidence of an illicit drug or a nonprescribed medication even though there were no obvious behavioral issues observed by providers.[42] These results were replicated in a study of 226 patients with chronic pain, which revealed that 46.5% of the sample taking prescribed opioids had abnormal urine toxicology screen results.[27] These studies suggest that risk assessment alone may not always identify patients who misuse pain medication and underscores the importance of regular urine toxicology screening along with behavioral observation and incorporation of self-report measures. Many clinics use immunoassay urine screens as the first line of analysis and then obtain results from GC/MS testing when it is important to detect the specific level of drug metabolite in the urine.

Prescription Drug Monitoring Programs

Potential solutions to the continuing rise in opioid abuse, misuse, and diversion have become an ongoing focus in regulatory, legal, and governmental action. Prescription Drug Monitoring Programs (PDMPs), one of the first diversion control tools established, monitor and analyze electronic prescription data transferred from pharmacies and practitioners. PDMPs are one facet of a universal precautions approach that has been implemented clinically over recent years. Universal precautions assume a degree of risk for each patient and includes risk assessment strategies as well as close patient monitoring in order to initiate and modify therapy in a safe and controlled manner. For instance, if a patient is screened and deemed to be at higher risk for opioid misuse, more frequent follow-up may be indicated as well as signing an opioid treatment agreement, prescribing fewer doses of opioids per prescription, requiring frequent urine screening, using pill counts, and regularly checking the PDMP. The goals of this plan also include an expansion of PDMPs among states and an objective to achieve consensus standards on the prescribing of opioids.

Instruments for Nonopioid Treatments

A number of instruments can be used to identify patients with problematic prescription drug use behaviors in the context of nonopioid treatments. Similar to the opioid-specific instruments that were described in previous sections (e.g., COMM, OCC), scores on these instruments may be taken as evidence of prescription drug misuse, but additional steps must be taken in order to diagnose patients with a prescription drug use disorder (i.e., prescription drug addiction). In the following sections, a brief description of some instruments that can be used to identify patients with problematic prescription drug use behaviors is provided. Although these instruments were not specifically developed and validated for patients with chronic pain, they have proven useful in clinical and research settings for the identification of patients with problematic prescription drug use behaviors and/or pharmacotherapy adherence issues.

The Drug Abuse Screening Test (DAST-10),[57] is a 10-item questionnaire that can be self-administered or administered by a trained interviewer. On the DAST-10, participants are asked to answer questions about illicit and prescription drug use over the past 12 months. The DAST-10 can be completed in less than 8 minutes. The DAST-10 is the shortened and most commonly used version of a 20-item DAST questionnaire (i.e., DAST-20). The Substance Abuse Subtle Screening Inventory (SASSI)[45] is a self-report questionnaire that can be used to assess substance use problems. The SASSI, which can be completed in 20 minutes, contains both subtle and face-valid items that were validated to assess the probability of having a substance use disorder. It also contains a validity scale to identify random responding and a defensiveness scale, which provides a measure of credibility of participants' reports of drug use. Also, the Drug Use Disorders Identification Test (DUDIT)[5] is an 11-item self-administered instrument designed to screen for drug-related problems. Items are based on the ICD-10 and DSM-IV diagnostic systems for substance abuse and dependence. A extended 54-item version (i.e., DUDIT-E) was recently developed and contains additional questions about drug-related consequences for individuals who have been identified as having a potential substance use disorder. Finally, the Alcohol, Smoking, and Substance Involvement Screening Test (NM-ASSIST) is a drug use screening instrument that can be used in general medical settings. The NM-ASSIST was developed by the National

Institutes on Drug Abuse in 2009 and was adapted from the World Health Organization ASSIST. The NM-ASSIST can be self-administered or completed by a trained interviewer. The NM-ASSIST can be easily scored and provides information about problematic use of substances used in the last three months. Responses on the NM-ASSIST generate a score suggesting the level of intervention needed and links to resources for conducting brief interventions and treatment referrals, if needed. Other instruments that can be used to screen for prescription drug use problems include the Adult Substance Use Survey,[68] the Triage Assessment for Addictive Disorder,[34] and the Benzodiazepine Dependence Questionnaire.[2]

IDENTIFYING PATIENTS WITH PRESCRIPTION DRUG ADDICTION

While the tools described here may be useful for identifying patients who are misusing prescription drugs over the course of therapy, the diagnosis of prescription drug addiction (e.g., opioid use disorder or sedative-hypnotic use disorder) can only be performed based on a clinical interview administered by a trained interviewer or clinician. For instance, the diagnosis of opioid addiction (i.e., opioid use disorder) has traditionally been based on the diagnostic criteria put forward by the American Psychiatric Association in the DSM. These criteria, however, have been criticized by many clinicians and researchers within the field of pain. For example, based on the DSM-IV, patients meeting criteria either for "opioid abuse" or "opioid dependence" were diagnosed with an opioid use disorder, and the blurred distinction between these two diagnoses created confusion for many clinicians. More important, only three criteria were needed in order to diagnose patients with opioid dependence based on the DSM-IV, and two of these criteria could include opioid tolerance and opioid withdrawal. Given that most patients are expected to show tolerance and/or withdrawal as a result of long-term opioid therapy, DSM-IV criteria were not considered suitable for patients with chronic pain prescribed opioids as they could lead to erroneous (i.e., false positive) diagnosis of opioid use disorder. Due to these criticisms, modifications were made in the fifth version of the DSM (DSM-5) that was published in 2013 for the diagnosis of opioid addiction. In the DSM-5, the distinction between opioid abuse and opioid dependence was abandoned, and diagnostic criteria from these two diagnoses are now combined to form a single disorder (i.e., opioid use disorder) of graded severity (i.e., mild, moderate, severe). Moreover, tolerance and withdrawal symptoms are no longer considered to be diagnostic criteria for individuals taking opioids (or any other substance) under medical supervision.

MANAGEMENT OF PATIENTS AT RISK OF NONADHERENCE OR PRESCRIPTION DRUG ADDICTION

A number of guidelines have been developed to facilitate the management of patients at risk of medication nonadherence (e.g., prescription drug misuse) or prescription drug addiction. Although some of these guidelines do address issues related to benzodiazepine use, they were primarily developed to minimize risks associated with opioid therapy.

The recommended gold standard of care for all patients considered for chronic opioid therapy includes a comprehensive assessment with a thorough history, a mandatory opioid agreement, and regular monitoring. For those patients at greatest risk for misuse of their medication, more frequent visits with urine toxicology screens, use of a compliance checklist, motivational counseling, and pill counts, if indicated, would be recommended,[14,29,41] Even though risk of opioid misuse and addiction remains, greater focus on risk screening and documentation of outcome is expected to help mitigate the misuse of prescription opioids.

Controlled-substance agreements have been used in clinics to document the expectations and roles of the patients and providers concerning the use of prescription opioids. The goal of these agreements is to use informed consent to address potential problems with opioid use and to improve patient compliance with opioid medication. Often, these documented agreements are used to educate the patients as well as inform patients of their responsibilities when using prescribed pain medication. An opioid therapy agreement identifies the conditions required of patients to be prescribed opioids for pain. Patients are often aware of the risks and complications associated with opioids, and termed conditions are needed to demonstrate that the patients are being responsible and benefiting from prescription opioids for pain. Typical sample conditions state that patients will (a) only use their prescribed medications as directed by their physician, (b) only receive prescription pain medication from one physician, (c) only use one pharmacy to fill prescriptions, (d) not receive additional medication if their prescription runs out early, (e) be unable to receive replacement medication if lost or stolen, (f) submit to periodic urine screens and pill counts to verify compliance, (g) be responsible in maintaining their appointments, (h) participate in all aspects of treatment (e.g., physical therapy, psychotherapy, and behavioral medicine), and (i) agree that if pain and daily function have not improved with their prescription pain medication, the physician has the right to taper the patient off the medication.

Each of the elements of the opioid therapy agreement should be clarified so patients know exactly what is expected of them. By signing the agreement, they are acknowledging their consent to the proposed treatment plan and agree to adhere to the specific conditions and responsibilities set by the clinic. It is recommended that each and every patient prescribed opioids for pain read and sign a controlled-substance agreement. Periodic use of an opioid compliance checklist can also be used to remind patients of their responsibilities when using opioids. For some, a violation of this agreement would mean tapering and eventually discontinuing prescription opioids. Unfortunately, violations of this agreement can go unreported, and often the treating physician has difficulty in tracking and verifying adherence.

A rational systematic approach in the treatment and management of chronic pain with opioid therapy, known as universal precautions, has received strong support from pain societies and clinicians alike.[31] This approach, borrowed from infectious disease paradigms, includes a means of identifying and monitoring patients at risk for misusing prescription opioids. Gourlay and colleagues[31] recommended the following steps when considering someone for chronic opioid therapy: (1) establish a diagnosis with the appropriate differential; (2) obtain a psychological assessment, including risk potential for addictive disorder; (3) complete an informed consent and treatment agreement; (4) assess level of pain and function; (5) begin an opioid therapy trial if indicated; (6) periodically reassess pain, function, and behavior (e.g., analgesia, activities of daily living, adverse events); (7) obtain at least annual urine screens; (8) review the primary diagnosis and comorbidities on every follow-up visit; and (9) thoroughly document all information. Additional evaluation and treatment planning can be provided by members of a comprehensive pain management center and communicated to the referring physicians. Some pain management specialists prefer to incorporate a trilateral agreement with the patient's primary care physician. After the patients have been followed by a pain specialist and stabilized on a particular opioid regimen, they may be referred back to the primary care provider. If issues of opioid noncompliance present themselves or there is a change in the pain diagnosis, the pain specialists could offer a reevaluation and consider additional treatments or changes in the medication regimen if necessary.

Despite the number of tools and management strategies available to clinicians for dealing with patients exhibiting problematic prescription drug use behaviors, experience tells us that some patients will continue to be noncompliant with treatment recommendations. In the context of opioid therapy, repeated violations of the opioid treatment agreement may be a sufficient condition for discontinuing opioids. If patients have become physically dependent on opioids, they should be tapered off their medication slowly to prevent opioid withdrawal. If opioid addiction is suspected, assessment by an addiction specialist and/or mental health professional should be mandated. Patients with an opioid addiction problem should be offered treatment both for pain and addiction, and opioid maintenance treatment offered through a licensed program (e.g., methadone maintenance center) may represent an appropriate avenue. If needed, opioid detoxification in a specialized inpatient or outpatient setting may be considered, but it is neither the standard of care nor supported by evidence for the management of chronic pain patients with prescription opioid addiction.

Interventions to Improve Adherence

Chronic pain patients who show evidence of noncompliance with prescription drugs are sometimes dismissed from clinic practice. Being "fired" from a clinic is not optimal since these patients often seek treatment elsewhere by going to the emergency department of a local hospital or engaging in illegal activity. A number of interventions have thus been recently developed in order to manage patients who show evidence of medication misuse over the course of pharmacotherapy. These interventions were primarily elaborated for patients prescribed long-term opioid therapy but could also be readily used for patients with adherence issues in the context of other pharmacological treatments.

Behavioral and Psychological Interventions

Evidence supporting the use of behavioral and psychological interventions to improve pharmacotherapy adherence among patients with pain has first been provided by Jamison and colleagues,[39] who conducted a randomized controlled trial examining the benefits of close monitoring and cognitive-behavioral interventions in order to improve opioid therapy adherence among high-risk patients. Close monitoring involved monthly urine screens as well as the use of opioid adherence checklists. Cognitive-behavioral interventions were designed to educate patients on opioid misuse and substance use problems, to enhance and maintain patients' motivation to be adherent with their prescribed opioid therapy regimen, to enhance patients' problem-solving skills, and to enhance patients' coping skills in order to deal with cravings and urges to misuse opioids. Results from their randomized controlled trial, which was conducted as part of a multidisciplinary pain program, showed that adherence training paired with careful monitoring of high-risk patients helped to reduce rates of prescription opioid misuse. In this trial, opioid adherence rates among high-risk patients were improved to that of low-risk patients. This encouraging study demonstrated the value and importance of risk assessment, frequent monitoring with monthly urine screens and opioid adherence checklists, and motivational counseling to help improve adherencewith opioids.

Support for the use of psychological interventions has also been provided by Garland et al.,[30] who conducted a randomized controlled trial examining the effectiveness of mindfulness-based interventions for improving adherence among patients prescribed long-term opioid therapy. In this trial, Mindfulness-Oriented Recovery Enhancement (MORE) was described as a novel multimodal intervention that integrates mindfulness training, cognitive reappraisal skills, and emotion regulation training. Patients were randomly assigned to either MORE or a support group. Results from the randomized controlled trial indicated that patients assigned to the eight-week MORE treatment condition reported significantly less opioid craving and opioid misuse behaviors at the end of the treatment than patients from the support group. This study provided preliminary support for the feasibility and effectiveness of MORE as a treatment for chronic pain patients exhibiting prescription opioid misuse behaviors.

Electronic Monitoring

Modern innovations, including the Internet and mobile technologies, offer significant opportunities to improve clinical outcomes and adherence to pharmacotherapy. Interactive and dynamic software programs that are designed to educate physicians, pharmacists, and patients will continue to be developed. Recently, there has been rapid growth of mobile health (m-health) and electronic health (e-health) applications in pain assessment and management.[4] The Global Observatory for eHealth of the World Health Organization defines m-health as "medical and public health practice supported by mobile/wireless devices, such as mobile phones, patient monitoring devices, tablets, personal digital assistants (PDAs), and wireless applications such as text messaging, downloadable programs (i.e., apps), movement monitors, and social media." The high density of mobile platforms worldwide now allow patients to access healthcare even where mobility, transportation requirements, or cost constraints present significant barriers to traditional face-to-face interactions with health care professionals.[21] These new technologies have increasingly become a viable option for managing patients with chronic pain conditions, and it is hoped that e-health and m-health applications will be used to improve clinical pain management outcomes and adherence to pharmacotherapy. With ever-expanding technology, larger segments of the population will have access to information and personal data designed to improve pain management, which hopefully will lead to reduced costs and more efficient healthcare utilization.

Surprisingly, despite recent technological advances, the interest in mobile technology for management of chronic pain has only recently started to develop, and there is still a paucity of large, high-quality trials to evaluate its efficacy. To date, the bulk of research on innovative technologies among patients with chronic pain has focused on the feasibility of these technologies for monitoring patients' levels of pain, physical activity, and mood.[8,38,58] Very little research, however, has been conducted among patients with pain to examine the effectiveness of technologies for improving adherence to pharmacotherapy. Technologies for improving pharmacotherapy adherence have been used among patients with other types of medical conditions, such as diabetes,[66] asthma,[59] hypertension,[19] and HIV.[33] Research will be needed to determine whether new technologies will eventually contribute to improving pharmacotherapy adherence among patients with chronic pain. Although electronic technologies will not completely replace the traditional face-to-face interaction with a healthcare professional, these interventions offer several promising benefits for monitoring and improving pharmacotherapy adherence.

CONCLUSIONS

Over the past few decades, pharmacotherapy has become the cornerstone of chronic pain management. Adherence to pharmacotherapy, however, is pivotal in order to optimize pain management outcomes and minimize potential risks associated with medication use. While adherence problems related to the use of benzodiazepines and headache medications are fairly prevalent among patients with pain conditions, rates of nonadherence associated with opioid therapy have recently become alarmingly high, both in primary care and tertiary care settings. Despite the potential benefits of opioids, some physicians remain uncomfortable or reluctant to prescribe opioids due to concerns related to prescription opioid misuse and addiction. There is nevertheless consensus that opioids can be safe and effective for carefully selected and monitored patients. Opioid risk assessment, using validated screening tools, is recommended for all patients who are being considered for long-term opioid therapy. For high-risk patients, such as those with high negative affect or psychiatric illness, the structure of opioid therapy may require more intensive monitoring, and comanagement with healthcare professionals specialized in addiction medicine or mental health may be necessary. While the nature and structure of therapy will vary from patient to patient, close attention to screening, monitoring, and documentation of opioid treatment outcomes will continue to be the gold standard of opioid therapy.

REFERENCES

1. Adams LL, Gatchel RJ, Robinson RC, et al. Development of a self-report screening instrument for assessing potential opioid medication misuse in chronic pain patients. *J Pain Symptom Manage.* 2004;27:440–459.
2. Baillie AJ, Mattick RP. The benzodiazepine dependence questionnaire: development, reliability and validity. *Brit J Psychiat.* 169:276–281, 1996
3. Belgrade MJ, Schamber CD, Lindgren BR. The DIRE score: predicting outcomes of opioid prescribing for chronic pain. *J Pain.* 2006;7:671–681.
4. Bender JL, Radhakrishnan A, Diorio C, Englesakis M, Jadad AR. Can pain be managed through the Internet? A systematic review of randomized controlled trials. *Pain.* 2011;152:1740–1750.
5. Berman AH, Palmstierna T, Kallmen H, Bergman H. The self-report Drug Use Disorders Identification Test: Extended (DUDIT-E): reliability, validity, and motivational index. *J Subst Abuse Treat.* 2007;32:357–369.
6. Boscarino JA, Rukstalis M, Hoffman SN, et al. Risk factors for drug dependence among out-patients on opioid therapy in a large US health-care system. *Addiction.* 2010;105:1776–1782.
7. Boscarino JA, Rukstalis MR, Hoffman SN, et al. Prevalence of prescription opioid-use disorder among chronic pain patients: comparison of the DSM-5 vs. DSM-4 diagnostic criteria. *J Addict Dis.* 2011;30:185–194.
8. Broderick JE, Schwartz JE, Schneider S, Stone AA. Can end-of-day reports replace momentary assessment of pain and fatigue? *J Pain.* 2009;10:274–281.
9. Butler SF, Budman SH, Fanciullo GJ, Jamison RN. Cross validation of the current opioid misuse measure to monitor chronic pain patients on opioid therapy. *Clin J Pain.* 2010;26:770–776.
10. Butler SF, Budman SH, Fernandez KC, Fanciullo GJ, Jamison RN. Cross-validation of a Screener to Predict Opioid Misuse in Chronic Pain Patients (SOAPP-R). *J Addict Med.* 2009;3:66–73.
11. Butler SF, Budman SH, Fernandez KC, et al. Development and validation of the Current Opioid Misuse Measure. *Pain.* 2007;130:144–156.
12. Butler SF, Fernandez K, Benoit C, Budman SH, Jamison RN. Validation of the revised Screener and Opioid Assessment for Patients with Pain (SOAPP-R). *J Pain.* 2008;9:360–372.

13. Calcaterra S, Glanz J, Binswanger IA. National trends in pharmaceutical opioid related overdose deaths compared to other substance related overdose deaths: 1999–2009. *Drug Alcohol Depend.* 2013;131:263–270.

14. Chou R, Fanciullo GJ, Fine PG, et al. Clinical guidelines for the use of chronic opioid therapy in chronic noncancer pain. *J Pain.* 2009;10:113–130.

15. Coambs RE, Jarry JL, Santhiapillai AC, Abrahamsohn RV, CM. A. The SISAP: a new screening instrument for identifying potential opioid abusers in the management of chronic nonmalignant pain in general medical practice. *Pain Res Manag.* 1996;1:155–162.

16. Colas R, Munoz P, Temprano R, Gomez C, Pascual J. Chronic daily headache with analgesic overuse: epidemiology and impact on quality of life. *Neurology.* 2004;62:1338–1342.

17. Compton PA, Wu SM, Schieffer B, Pham Q, Naliboff BD. Introduction of a self-report version of the Prescription Drug Use Questionnaire and relationship to medication agreement noncompliance. *J Pain Symptom Manage.* 2008;36:383–395.

18. Cupini LM, De Murtas M, Costa C, et al. Obsessive-compulsive disorder and migraine with medication-overuse headache. *Headache.* 2009;49:1005–1013.

19. Da Costa FA, Guerreiro JP, De Melo MN, Miranda AC, Martins AP. Effect of reminder cards on compliance with antihypertensive medication. *Int J Pharm Pract.* 2005;13:205–211.

20. Darnall BD, Stacey BR. Sex differences in long-term opioid use: cautionary notes for prescribing in women. *Arch Intern Med.* 2012;172:431–432.

21. Dayer L, Heldenbrand S, Anderson P, Gubbins PO, Martin BC. Smartphone medication adherence apps: potential benefits to patients and providers. *J Am Pharm Assoc.* 2013;53:172–181.

22. Dersh J, Gatchel RJ, Mayer T, Polatin P, Temple OR. Prevalence of psychiatric disorders in patients with chronic disabling occupational spinal disorders. *Spine.* 2006;31:1156–1162.

23. Drummond DC. Theories of drug craving, ancient and modern. *Addiction.* 2001;96:33–46.

24. Dunn KM, Saunders KW, Rutter CM, et al. Opioid prescriptions for chronic pain and overdose: a cohort study. *Ann Intern Med.* 2010;152:85–92.

25. Edlund MJ, Sullivan M, Steffick D, Harris KM, Wells KB. Do users of regularly prescribed opioids have higher rates of substance use problems than nonusers? *Pain Med.* 2007;8:647–656.

26. Edlund MJ, Sullivan MD, Han X, Booth BM. Days with pain and substance use disorders: is there an association? *Clin J Pain.* 2013;29:689–695.

27. Fishbain DA, Cutler RB, Rosomoff HL, Rosomoff RS. Validity of self-reported drug use in chronic pain patients. *Clin J Pain.* 1999;15:184–191.

28. Fleming MF, Balousek SL, Klessig CL, Mundt MP, Brown DD. Substance use disorders in a primary care sample receiving daily opioid therapy. *J Pain.* 2007;8:573–582.

29. Furlan AD, Reardon R, Weppler C. Opioids for chronic noncancer pain: a new Canadian practice guideline. *Can Med Assoc J.* 2010;182:923–930.

30. Garland EL, Manusov EG, Froeliger B, Kelly A, Williams JM, Howard MO. Mindfulness-oriented recovery enhancement for chronic pain and prescription opioid misuse: results from an early-stage randomized controlled trial. *J Consult Clin Psychol.* 2014;82:448–459.

31. Gourlay DL, Heit HA, Almahrezi A. Universal precautions in pain medicine: a rational approach to the treatment of chronic pain. *Pain Med.* 2005;6:107–112.

32. Gudin JA, Mogali S, Jones JD, Comer SD. Risks, management, and monitoring of combination opioid, benzodiazepines, and/or alcohol use. *Postgrad Med.* 2013;125:115–130.

33. Hardy H, Kumar V, Doros G, et al. Randomized controlled trial of a personalized cellular phone reminder system to enhance adherence to antiretroviral therapy. *AIDS Patient Care STDs.* 2011;25:153–161.

34. Hoffmann NG. *Triage Assessment for Addictive Disorders.* Smithfield, RI: Evince Clinical Assessments; 1996.

35. Hojsted J, Nielsen PR, Guldstrand SK, Frich L, Sjogren P. Classification and identification of opioid addiction in chronic pain patients. *Eur J Pain.* 2010;14:1014–1020.

36. Jamison RN, Edwards RR. Risk factor assessment for problematic use of opioids for chronic pain. *Clin Neuropsychol.* 2013;27:60–80.

37. Jamison RN, Martel MO, Huang CC, Jurcik D, Edwards RR. Efficacy of the Opioid Compliance Checklist to Monitor Chronic Pain Patients on Opioid Therapy in Primary Care. *J Pain.* 2016;17(4):414–423.

38. Jamison RN, Raymond SA, Levine JG, Slawsby EA, Nedeljkovic SS, Katz NP. Electronic diaries for monitoring chronic pain: 1-year validation study. *Pain.* 2001;91:277–285.

39. Jamison RN, Ross EL, Michna E, Chen LQ, Holcomb C, Wasan AD. Substance misuse treatment for high-risk chronic pain patients on opioid therapy: a randomized trial. *Pain.* 2010;150:390–400.

40. Jones JD, Mogali S, Comer SD. Polydrug abuse: a review of opioid and benzodiazepine combination use. *Drug Alcohol Dep.* 2012;125:8–18.

41. Kahan M, Mailis-Gagnon A, Tunks E. Canadian guideline for safe and effective use of opioids for chronic non-cancer pain: implications for pain physicians. *Pain Res Manag.* 2011;16:157–158.

42. Katz NP, Sherburne S, Beach M, et al. Behavioral monitoring and urine toxicology testing in patients receiving long-term opioid therapy. *Anesth Analg.* 2003;97:1097–1102.

43. Kouyanou K, Pither CE, Wessely S. Medication misuse, abuse and dependence in chronic pain patients. *J Psychosom Res.* 1997;43:497–504.

44. Lauwerier E, Paemeleire K, Van Damme S, Goubert L, Crombez G. Medication use in patients with migraine and medication-overuse headache: the role of problem-solving and attitudes about pain medication. *Pain.* 2011;152:1334–1339.

45. Lazowski LE, Miller FG, Boye MW, Miller GA. Efficacy of the Substance Abuse Subtle Screening Inventory-3 (SASSI-3) in identifying substance dependence disorders in clinical settings. *J Pers Assess.* 1998;71:114–128.

46. Liebschutz JM, Saitz R, Weiss RD, et al. Clinical factors associated with prescription drug use disorder in urban primary care patients with chronic pain. *J Pain.* 2010;11:1047–1055.

47. Lintzeris N, Mitchell TB, Bond AJ, Nestor L, Strang J. Pharmacodynamics of diazepam co-administered with methadone or buprenorphine under high dose conditions in opioid dependent patients. *Drug Alcohol Dep.* 2007;91:187–194.

48. Manchikanti L, Giordano J, Boswell MV, Fellows B, Manchukonda R, Pampati V. Psychological factors as predictors of opioid abuse and illicit drug use in chronic pain patients. *J Opiod Manag.* 2007;3:89–100.

49. Martel MO, Dolman AJ, Edwards RR, Jamison RN, Wasan AD. The association between negative affect and prescription opioid misuse in patients with chronic pain: the mediating role of opioid craving. *J Pain.* 2014;15:90–100.

50. Martel MO, Wasan AD, Jamison RN, Edwards RR. Catastrophic thinking and increased risk for prescription opioid misuse in patients with chronic pain. *Drug Alcohol Dep.* 2013;132:335–341.

51. Michna E, Jamison RN, Pham LD, et al. Urine toxicology screening among chronic pain patients on opioid therapy: frequency and predictability of abnormal findings. *Clin J Pain.* 2007;23:173–179.

52. Nielsen S, Lintzeris N, Bruno R, et al. Benzodiazepine use among chronic pain patients prescribed opioids: associations with pain, physical and mental health, and health service utilization. *Pain Med.* 2015;16:356–366.

53. Passik SD, Kirsh KL, Whitcomb L, et al. Monitoring outcomes during long-term opioid therapy for noncancer pain: results with the Pain Assessment and Documentation Tool. *J Opiod Manag.* 2005;1:257–266.

54. Radat F, Chanraud S, Di Scala G, Dousset V, Allard M. Psychological and neuro-psychological correlates of dependence-related behaviour in medication overuse headaches: a one year follow-up study. *J Headache Pain.* 2013;14:59.

55. Rossi P, Faroni JV, Nappi G. Medication overuse headache: predictors and rates of relapse in migraine patients with low medical needs. A 1-year prospective study. *Cephalalgia.* 2008;28:1196–1200.

56. Saunders KW, Von Korff M, Campbell CI, et al. Concurrent use of alcohol and sedatives among persons prescribed chronic opioid therapy: prevalence and risk factors. *J Pain.* 2012;13:266–275.

57. Skinner HA. The drug abuse screening test. *Addict Behav.* 1982;7:363–371.

58. Stone AA, Broderick JE, Schwartz JE, Shiffman S, Litcher-Kelly L, Calvanese P. Intensive momentary reporting of pain with an electronic diary: reactivity, compliance, and patient satisfaction. *Pain.* 2003;104:343–351.

59. Strandbygaard U, Thomsen SF, Backer V. A daily SMS reminder increases adherence to asthma treatment: a three-month follow-up study. *Respir Med.* 2010;104:166–171.

60. Straube A, Pfaffenrath V, Ladwig KH, et al. Prevalence of chronic migraine and medication overuse headache in Germany—the German DMKG headache study. *Cephalalgia.* 2010;30:207–213.

61. Sullivan M. Clarifying opioid misuse and abuse. *Pain.* 2013;154:2239–2240.

62. Tiffany ST, Wray JM. The clinical significance of drug craving. *Ann NY Acad Sci.* 2012;1248:1–17.

63. Tragesser SL, Jones RE, Robinson RJ, Stutler A, Stewart A. Borderline personality disorder features and risk for prescription opioid use disorders. *J Pers Disord.* 2013;27:427–441.

64. Turk DC, Swanson KS, Gatchel RJ. Predicting opioid misuse by chronic pain patients: a systematic review and literature synthesis. *Clin J Pain.* 2008;24:497–508.

65. Verdejo-Garcia A, Lawrence AJ, Clark L. Impulsivity as a vulnerability marker for substance-use disorders: review of findings from high-risk research, problem gamblers and genetic association studies. *Neurosci Biobehav Rev.* 2008;32:777–810.

66. Vervloet M, Linn AJ, van Weert JC, de Bakker DH, Bouvy ML, van Dijk L. The effectiveness of interventions using electronic reminders to improve adherence to chronic medication: a systematic review of the literature. *J Am Med Inform Assoc.* 2012;19:696–704.

67. Vowles KE, McEntee ML, Julnes PS, Frohe T, Ney JP, van der Goes DN. Rates of opioid misuse, abuse, and addiction in chronic pain: a systematic review and data synthesis. *Pain.* 2015;156:569–576.

68. Wanberg KW. *The Adult Substance Use Survey (ASUS)*. Arvada, CO: Center for Addictions Research and Evaluation; 1997.
69. Wasan AD, Butler SF, Budman SH, Benoit C, Fernandez K, Jamison RN. Psychiatric history and psychologic adjustment as risk factors for aberrant drug-related behavior among patients with chronic pain. *Clin J Pain*. 2007;23:307–315.
70. Wasan AD, Butler SF, Budman SH, et al. Does report of craving opioid medication predict aberrant drug behavior among chronic pain patients? *Clin J Pain*. 2009;25:193–198.
71. Wasan AD, Ross EL, Michna E, et al. Craving of prescription opioids in patients with chronic pain: a longitudinal outcomes trial. *J Pain*. 2012;13:146–154.
72. Webster LR. Considering the risks of benzodiazepines and opioids together. *Pain Med*. 2010;11:801–802.
73. Webster LR, Cochella S, Dasgupta N, et al. An analysis of the root causes for opioid-related overdose deaths in the United States. *Pain Med*. 2011;12 Suppl 2:S26–35.
74. Webster LR, Webster RM. Predicting aberrant behaviors in opioid-treated patients: preliminary validation of the Opioid Risk Tool. *Pain Med*. 2005;6:432–442.
75. Wilsey BL, Fishman SM, Tsodikov A, Ogden C, Symreng I, Ernst A. Psychological comorbidities predicting prescription opioid abuse among patients in chronic pain presenting to the emergency department. *Pain Med*. 2008;9:1107–1117.
76. Wu SM, Compton P, Bolus R, et al. The Addiction Behaviors Checklist: validation of a new clinician-based measure of inappropriate opioid use in chronic pain. *J Pain Symptom Manage*. 2006;32:342–351.

CHAPTER 4

cVɔ

The Use of Drug Testing in Promoting Treatment Adherence in Pain Medicine

DOUGLAS L. GOURLAY AND HOWARD A. HEIT

INTRODUCTION

Urine drug testing (UDT) is a key recommended component of risk evaluation and mitigation strategies in the clinical care of patients prescribed controlled substances for chronic pain treatment, but there is little hard evidence in the literature to support its effectiveness in improving therapeutic outcomes or reducing misuse, abuse, diversion, or opioid-related morbidity or mortality.

In fact, one of the core concepts of risk management, the so-called universal precautions approach has been misinterpreted to imply "mandatory urine drug testing for everyone."[1] Urine drug testing is mentioned only once in the paper that suggested universal precautions approach to pain medicine,[2] and UDT was intended to be just one additional tool among many others to considered in the evaluation of *all patients*, rather than relying on a clinician's subjective impression of risk in any given case. To be clear, the centerpiece to a universal precautions approach to risk management is not UDT. Although UDT may play an important part, the real value in a universal precautions approach is to consider risk in a comprehensive way and as an inherent aspect of human behavior. "If you have a pulse, you have a risk" is an important concept to consider in the context of several medical settings, including chronic pain management.[3]

The notion of trust and trustworthiness in pain management has been examined in some detail by Buchman et al.[4] While a qualitative study, using semistructured interviews in an urban setting in British Columbia, the authors outline the challenges both for patients and practitioners in decision-making in situations where there is all too frequently a less than complete data set. The impact that these realities have on the therapeutic relationship between clinician and patient can be significant. Ideally, this impact is positive, but more often than not it is likely to be destructive to the therapeutic relationship.[5]

Krishnamurthy et al.[6] have also examined the effect of drug testing in an academic pain center. They conducted a retrospective cohort comparison of patients who were and who were not subjected to an initial UDT and found that drug testing was associated with increased no-show and dropout rates from the clinic.[6] While this paper raises many interesting and as yet unanswered questions about the role of drug testing in patient care, it brings up an overarching concern and question about where patients who have substance use disorders (SUDs) go when they drop out from treatment. The implication is that this is neither good for the patient nor the society that is left to deal them.

Unfortunately, the rise in prescription-opioid deaths has led to more of a reactive than hypothesis-driven approach to curbing this public health crisis.[7–9] The response to this epidemic has been more through regulation than a carefully balanced educational or well-constructed preventative approach, following validated public-health principles.[10] In this regard, mandatory drug testing is taking center stage as the tool to address this problem despite a striking paucity of scientific evidence to support the practice.

There is also a clear potential for abuse through drug testing. This abuse is not simply financial, rewarding clinics and laboratories, but there is an appreciable opportunity cost that impacts patients who must disrupt their lives to undergo these tests.

Starrels et al.[11] reviewed the effects treatment agreements and UDT on reducing opioid misuse and concluded that neither practice, at the present time, could be supported by evidence-based medicine. Notwithstanding this absence of a high level of empirical proof, it is our experienced-based opinion that treatment agreements and UDT are valuable clinical tools when used in a clearly patient-centered fashion.[12] And many authoritative guidelines are mandating or strongly recommending that UDT be a "standard of care" with respect to the use of chronic opioids.[13]

With these conditions and considerations in mind, we utilize case-based examples to frame UDT and other strategies for improving treatment adherence in the context of "best clinical practices."

IS UDT WARRANTED?

It might seem obvious that a chapter built on a foundation of universal precautions and adherence in pain treatment with opioids would recommend drug testing for everyone—but we do not believe that this is always a foregone conclusion. The first question to ask and answer when considering any universal (default) practice is: "What is the value to the patient?"[14]

Since UDT is only one tool in the clinician's proverbial toolbox, and since there is no proof that its use leads to desirable therapeutic outcomes, should this tool be applied irrespective of individual patient context or circumstances?

From the outset, we should state that UDT in and of itself is relatively limited in its ability to provide definitive answers to all but a few questions clinicians would expect or hope these tests would answer. It does, however provide the basis for a useful differential diagnosis and may become the stepping-off point for a clinical discussion with the patient that otherwise might have been very difficult to initiate.

For example, UDT is not able to independently corroborate important diagnoses such as physical dependency or addiction.[15] The presence or absence of any given analyte may be suggestive, but it is just that—a laboratory result that must be interpreted in the overall clinical context.

UDT is also not able to inform a clinician if a patient is diverting prescribed medications, nor is it able to tell if the patient is taking more or less medication than has been prescribed.[15] Historically, it was thought that accurate relationships between dose taken and quantified UDT results obtained exist[16] and could help clinicians know if their patient was adherent (taking medications only as directed). This hoped-for relationship has not been found to be quantitatively reliable. The drug that can be abused most easily, from a UDT perspective, is the one that is legitimately present in the urine sample.[14]

The factors that takes UDT out of a forensic context or potentially adversarial clinician–patient mode and moves it into the therapeutic relational realm is contextual interpretation and communication. Patient-centered UDT is defined by the manner and means by which UDT is introduced and those actions taken in response to the UDT results, not merely by the fact that a urine sample was collected and the results were documented in the medical record. Since the end outcome of any risk evaluation and mitigation strategy is to reduce harm—not simply demonstrate strict obeisance to a regulatory requirement or standard—then UDT can be a value "commodity" of communication, education, and strengthening of the therapeutic relationship, both in monitoring and in improving adherence to an indicated medication regimen involving potentially toxic drugs.

So what are the correct motivational ingredients to consider in order to optimize UDT in one's practice? The first might be one's commitment to risk management. Putting a UDT program in place as part of a clinical care plan is a very visible commitment to addressing patient as well as public safety with respect to the prescription of controlled substances. It remains one of the few objective tests available in an otherwise largely subjective clinical domain. Since it has become repeatedly demonstrated that a significant proportion of even very well-intended patients do not use prescribed medications of any type exactly as directed, UDT is simply a means of measuring something that matters a lot. And, in so doing, it may plant a seed in the minds of patients to reinforce adherence, strengthening good intentions and supporting both therapeutic and safe behaviors.

Another reason is to remind patients who have struggled in the past with prescription or other drug use problems that the clinician is as committed to their recovery as they are. Again, asking the question is important, but what one does with the results remains key and is our focus going forward.

Finally, there is certainly a regulatory commitment to the use of UDT in clinical care as part of a comprehensive strategy of risk management. The lack of literature to support this notwithstanding, it is important to remain within regulatory and medical board guidelines in one's practice.

Medical Necessity

Some clinicians have been encouraged to add UDT to their practices as a means of increasing revenues in an era of declining reimbursement for core clinical services. The explosion of the pain management laboratory industry has led to a dramatic increase in both laboratory as well as office-based drug testing. It is now possible to have sophisticated liquid chromatography (LC)–mass spectrometry (MS)/MS instrumentation in the form of desktop analyzers in private practitioners' offices. In fact, these schemes are often being met with third-party billing investigations that in some cases have led to criminal prosecutions for fraudulent billing.[17] Even in high-risk patient populations, clinicians *can* test too frequently.[14]

Clearly, when the decision to order a test directly rewards the ordering practitioner, there is an inherent conflict of interest, with a significant risk of these tests being ordered unnecessarily and excessively (i.e., without specific medical necessity).[18] Equally, the more tests one orders, the more test result data must be interpreted, documented, and managed. This creates significant risk of missing critically important, and clinically actionable data can get lost in a sea of "noise."

Perhaps the first thing to ask is: What is a medically necessary test? As a practical definition, for a test to be medically necessary and clinical relevant it must contain three basic elements. The first addresses whether it will aid in diagnosis or treatment, answering the query, "Why the test was ordered?" To be medically necessary, there must be a clinical question that the ordered test can reasonably be expected to answer. With respect to UDT, the questions "What medications is this patient actually taking?" or "Is this patient only taking the medications I have prescribed?" fit into this category.

The second element addresses timeliness, appropriate responsiveness, and management of the results of the test, answering the query, "What result was obtained, was there an indication for a change in diagnosis or treatment with a plan for timely and adequate communication to the patient and other stakeholder clinicians, and were these thought processes appropriately recorded in the chart?" Simply ordering a test without doing anything with the results is clearly not clinically relevant and renders the test medically unnecessary.

Finally, there must be a clinically actionable step taken, properly documented in the medical record, that is consistent with the results obtained and describes the clinical course and follow-up plan. In cases of results that support the assessment of clinical stability, "staying the course" is a completely acceptable action.

Clearly, to be medically necessary implies a degree of clinical relevance that may be difficult to demonstrate unless there is a well-structured, consistent, and rational clinic policy. While it might be appropriate to recommend an initial test for all patients, and retest on some periodic basis, testing as a whole must be tied to some initial or ongoing assessment of risk. The simple act of ordering a drug test and collecting a sample for analysis has not been shown to be of any therapeutic value. When the decision to test remunerates the ordering clinician in the absence of such clinical relevance, it becomes very difficult to refute the initial assessment that financial gain was the prime motivator in ordering UDT.

CHOOSING A LABORATORY

At the present time, there are an enormous number of laboratories and device manufacturers competing for the opportunity to perform clinical testing for pain management clinicians. So what should one look for in a testing laboratory? Clearly, it is important to have confidence in the lab's methodology and scientific accuracy.[19] To this end, the current lack of uniform formal proficiency testing in the field of pain management laboratory testing presents a problem. With time, regulatory oversight for these labs will ensure that all clinical labs exist and function on a level playing field. One measure of potential credibility is to ensure that the lab is certified by the Clinical Laboratory Improvement Amendments (CLIA). In parallel with laboratory certification, the Center for Medicare and Medicaid Services has begun the process of establishing specific reimbursement parameters to avoid excessive billing for drug testing.

For the most part, nationally represented, CLIA-certified labs with a proven track record in the field should be one's first choice. These labs tend to have a well-established infrastructure of sample collection, analysis, and result reporting in place, which simplifies the process of drug testing for the clinician. Rapid turnaround (time from sample receipt to reporting) should be 48 hours or less.[14]

In some cases, these labs engage in proficiency testing, which often involves externally validated sample analysis that can be compared against known results to ensure both accuracy and reliability in terms of methodologies used.

Dangers of Scientific Overreach

One of the particularly dangerous aspects of drug testing is the sometimes unsubstantiated claims made by certain labs in terms of their ability to reliably detect nonadherence with prescribed dosing schedules of controlled substances. Typically, these labs compare a patient's results with descriptive statistics from "known compliant" patient populations but without contextual (inter- and intraindividual variability) validation.

At the present time, there are no scientific means of relating amount of drug taken and amount recovered from UDT samples. Further, the notion that there is a "known compliant" patient database somewhere is flawed in many different ways.[14] The only persons who could possibly know if patients are "completely adherent" with prescribed medications are the patients themselves. The literature is quite clear that self-report alone is a very unreliable metric when trying to assess aberrant behavior.[20] In fact, there may be a significant number of patients who genuinely believe they are following their doctors' instructions to the letter despite the fact that on closer examination their medication use is anything but adherent. The following case demonstrates this point.

A young health professional (physiotherapist) was assessed for problematic use of immediate-release, short-acting oxycodone tablets. The patient complained of significant withdrawal-related pain (end of dose failure) over the course of 24 hours, culminating upon waking in the morning hours. Amplified or recurrent pain due to inadequate sustained analgesic levels is typically addressed through the addition of controlled-release medications. To this end, she was started on an appropriate dose of controlled-release oxycodone, dose adjusted for the antici-pated improved analgesic response due to the twice-daily dosing schedule.

Despite this change, she continued to complain of withdrawal-mediated pain. The dose was increased, and the frequency of dosing was adjusted to three times daily. Her total daily dose increased but clinical stability was not improved.

It became apparent that more details about how the patient was actually tak-ing her medication were needed. She assured her prescriber that she was tak-ing the medications three times per day. Unfortunately, she was taking them at 9 AM, 10 AM, and 11 AM! There was no intent to mislead or deceive, simply a misunderstanding of what her prescriber meant by "three times daily dosing." In this patient's mind, hourly dosing made perfect sense, since that was her per-ceived duration of action for this drug.

One of the most important benefits of working closely with a testing laboratory is the ability to call and speak with someone who can help inter-pret apparently anomalous results. That said, it is important to realize that a scientifically "accurate" result might not always translate into a clinically useful piece of information.

When unexpected results appear on a patient's laboratory report form, it is important to consider the overall clinical context for that patient. An otherwise clinically stable patient with an unexpected negative UDT result for a prescribed medication may, at first blush, appear as evidence of mis-behavior or drug diversion. It is certainly important that clinicians be pre-pared to reassess their evaluation of "clinical stability." It is also important to remember that analyte recovery rates from samples vary, depending on methodologies used and analyte(s) tested for. As such, a drug with rela-tively low recovery rates may be reported as "not detected" when in fact the patient was taking the drug exactly as prescribed.

As an example, a known population of buprenorphine users was found to have an unexpectedly large number of negative UDT samples for this target drug. These were "known" users because they were part of a buprenorphine maintenance treatment program where most were engaged in observed dosing. When the lab was contacted in this regard, the scientific director advised that due to a relatively low buprenorphine/norbuprenorphine recovery rate from the donor sample, it was very possible that the reports of "not detected" in patients known to be using this drug represented a scientifically correct result but a result that was completely misleading from a clinical perspective. In fact, it has been reported in the literature that LC-MS/MS has a sensitivity issue with respect to buprenorphine and its metabolites.[21]

Point of Care Versus Laboratory Testing

Not all drug testing occurs in a laboratory. Some tests are conducted at the point of sample collection. These tests are often referred to as "test cups" or "test strips" and generally fall into the category of "presumptive testing."

To be clear, the nomenclature of drug testing is undergoing a change. Where the forensic literature was replete with statements of "screens" and "confirmatory" testing, we now talk about "presumptive" and "definitive" testing in clinical care.[14]

In presumptive testing, methods are used that tend to identify classes of drugs rather than individual drugs or drug metabolites. These analytes are not specifically identified but rather are indirectly identified, typically through immunoassay methodologies.[14] In the interests of providing rapid results, there is often a significant price to be paid in terms of accuracy and reliability.

Take, for example, the "opiate" immunoassay test. (Table 4.1) This immunoassay reagent is actually targeted toward the morphine and codeine molecules. Sensitivity toward semisynthetic or synthetic agents is unreliable in

Table 4.1. SOURCES OF APLOID ANALGESIC

Natural (Extracted from Opium)	Semisynthetic (Derived from Opium Extracts)	Synthetic (Manufactured)
• Codeine	• Hydrocodone	• Meperidine
• Morphine	• Oxycodone	• Fentanyl family
• Thebaine	• Hydromorphone	• Methadone
	• Oxymorphone	• Tapentadol
	• Buprenorphine	

the first case and nonexistent in the latter case.[22] If the pretest probability of drug detection is low, and all we are looking for are morphine/codeine/heroin users, this can be a very effective test. This was the case in traditional regulated testing where the vast majority of sample donors (i.e., the workforce) were correctly expected to be nonusers.

Unfortunately, the immunoassay tests have a very high incidence of false positives (and, in some cases, false negatives) for these and other analytes.[23] So, in a non-drug using donor who is prescribed a quinolone antibiotic, a false "opiate positive" immunoassay result is not at all uncommon. (Table 4.2) Of course, definitive testing will be able to rule out this false positive, but only if the interpreting clinician is aware of this interaction and is alert enough to order the definitive test.

Table 4.2. EXAMPLES OF POTENTIAL FALSE POSITIVES DUE TO CROSS-REACTING COMPOUNDS FOR CERTAIN IMMUNOASSAYS

Immunoassay Affected[a]	Cross-Reacting Drug[b]
Opiates	Quinolone antibiotics (e.g., levofloxacin, ofloxacin)[96,97]
Buprenorphine Tramadol	Analgesic[114]
Fentanyl; MDMA (Ecstasy), amphetamine	Trazodone (antidepressant)[98,102,111,116]
Benzodiazepine, LSD	Sertraline (antidepressant)[118,119]
Methadone	Quetiapine (atypical antipsychotic)[105]
Methadone	Tapentadol (analgesic)[121]
PCP	Venlafaxine (antidepressant)[100,103]
PCP	Dextromethorphan (antitussive)[108]
PCP	Tramadol (analgesic)[109,123]
PCP	Lamotrigine (anticonvulsant)[120]
Amphetamine	Selegiline (for Parkinson's disease)[99]
Amphetamine	Promethazine (for allergies, agitation, nausea, vomiting)[107]
Amphetamine	l-methamphetamine (over-the-counter nasal inhaler)[14]
Amphetamine	Pseudoephedrine (over-the-counter decongestant)[115]
Amphetamine	Bupropion (antidepressant)[104]
Amphetamine	Ranitidine (histamine H2-receptor antagonist)[112]
Fentanyl	Risperidone (antipsychotic)[113]
THCA, benzodiazepine	Efavirenz (antiretroviral)[101,106,122]
THCA	Proton pump inhibitors (e.g., pantoprazole)[110]

Note: LSD = lysergic acid diethylamide; MDMA = 3,4-methylenedioxymethamphetamine; PCP = phencyclidine; THCA = delta-9-tetrahydrocannabinol-9-carboxylic acid.
[a] Only some immunoassays are affected; cross-reactivity patterns change constantly as reagents are refined to address these issues. [b] Or metabolite of the drug.

However, point of care testing has found considerable utility in the drug treatment setting where the immediacy of knowing test results can outweigh the potential false positives associated with this technique. Outside of the forensic world, all immunoassay results do not need to be "confirmed" by a second scientific method. Only those results that are contested, or where are other indicia of concern, need to undergo further testing.

In the pain management population who are actively being prescribed opioids, immunoassay testing has considerable limitations. First, the pretest probability of use (i.e., of prescribed medications) is exceedingly high; in fact, the absence of a controlled substance in the donor sample may cause as much concern as the presence of a nonprescribed drug. The difference lies in the "legitimacy" of the analytes presence in the donor sample.

As a general rule, the pain management community will find less use in simple, immunoassay testing methods ("presumptive testing") compared to the general population as a whole. Part of the reason for this rests in a simple assessment of pretest probability of the population under study. For the most part, the general population is not expected to be positive for common immunoassay drugs of abuse. In contrast, the pain community will typically have a very high incidence of legitimate prescription opioid use. This limits the utility of a simple immunoassay identification system. In the monitoring of prescription drug users, we are interested in the sample being positive for the appropriate class of drug but also positive for the specific member of that class.

A good example to illustrate this point is the pain patient who is prescribed transdermal fentanyl to manage pain. An immunoassay opiate test that is positive or negative says very little about clinical stability of this patient, since a negative test result is entirely consistent with a fentanyl-using donor. Fentanyl, a synthetic opioid, is not detected by opiate immunoassay testing.[14] On the other hand, a positive result might be a result of a recent antibiotic cross-reactivity, but it might also be a result of illicit/unprescribed drug use. More definitive testing (which probably should have been done from the outset) is likely necessary, unless the patient volunteers information that resolves the dilemma.

In fact, the current debate rages between individually ordered test elements and what in the industry are commonly referred to as "drug panel" testing. (Table 4.3) The fact is that we are unable to discern, with certainty, who is or is not using drugs inappropriately. More importantly, we can't divine which drug or drugs a person might be using if they are non-adherent.

Table 4.3. EXAMPLE OF DRUGS/METABOLITES COMMONLY
DETECTED IN A PAIN MANAGEMENT PANEL

Drug or Drug Class	Drugs and/or METABOLITES[a] included
Amphetamines	Amphetamine
	Methamphetamine
	MDMA (Ecstasy)
	MDEA (Eve)
	MDA
	Phentermine
Barbiturates	Butalbital
	Phenobarbital
Benzodiazepines	Alprazolam
	Clonazepam
	Diazepam
	Flurazepam
	Lorazepam
	Nordiazepam
	Oxazepam
	Temazepam
Cocaine	Benzoylecgonine
Heroin	Heroin (diacetylmorphine)
	6-MAM
	6-acetylcodeine
Marijuana	THCA
Opioids	Buprenorphine
	Norbuprenorphine
	Codeine
	Norcodeine
	Dihydrocodeine
	Fentanyl
	Norfentanyl
	Hydrocodone
	Norhydrocodone
	Hydromorphone
	Meperidine
	Normeperidine
	Methadone
	EDDP
	Morphine

(continued)

	Table 4.3. CONTINUED
Drug or Drug Class	Drugs and/or METABOLITES[a] included
	Oxycodone
	Noroxycodone
	Oxymorphone
	Tapentadol
	Tramadol
	O-desmethyl-tramadol
	N-desmethyl-tramadol
PCP	PCP
Carisoprodol	Carisoprodol
	Meprobamate
Anticonvulsants	Gabapentin
	Pregabalin

Note: 6-MAM = 6-monoacetylmorphine; EDDP = 2-ethylidene-1,5-dimethyl-3,3-diphenylpyrrolidine; MDMA = 3,4-methylenedioxymethamphetamine; MDA = 3,4-methylenedioxyamphetamine; MDEA = 3,4-methylenedioxyethylamphetamine; PCP = phencyclidine; THCA = delta-9-tetrahydrocannabinol-9-carboxylic acid.
[a]For some drugs that are rapidly metabolized, the metabolites may be more important than testing for the parent drug.

INTRODUCING DRUG TESTING INTO YOUR PRACTICE

One of the more common communication issues clinicians struggle with is how to broach the issue of drug testing with patients in clinical care (Box 4.1). The overwhelming feeling is that drug testing will be seen as intrusive and mistrustful.[24,25] Some have expressed concerns that they feel like they are judging the patient or the patient's lifestyle. To a certain extent, this all can be true unless steps are taken to address these concerns.

Regarding the issue of "judging" the patient, this is unquestionably true. The practice of medicine involves a good deal of judging of information and data, but all judgments must be made with the patient's health and privacy in the forefront and as the motivating factor.

Take glycemic control as an example. When managing diabetics using insulin to control their blood glucose levels, patients are typically expected to record their blood glucose levels and report this back to the treating clinician. If a patient reports that his or her glycemic control has been "good," we typically still follow with a periodic HbA1c to support this assertion of good control.[3] The test is not ordered because we do not trust the patient but rather because we know that the information

---

Box 4.1

TALKING TO PATIENTS ABOUT UDT

EXAMPLE 1: NEW PATIENT

Clinician	"One of the things that we offer our patients with chronic pain is urine drug testing. This is a safe and effective means of assisting with risk management, and it is part of our commitment to you as the patient to ensure optimum care."
Patient	"Oh, so you mean I don't have to do it?"
Clinician	"Of course you don't have to do it, but you need to understand that failure to take advantage of this test may limit the options that I can safely offer you in terms of medication management."

EXAMPLE 2: EXISTING PATIENTᴬ

Clinician	"Urine drug testing is a safe and cost-effective method of helping to manage risk in order to make sure that I'm here next week, next month, or next year when you need me and to make sure that you get the care you need."
Patient	"Do you think that I have a drug problem?"
Clinician	"I don't necessarily think that you have a drug problem, but in the interest of fairness and balance, testing is something that is now being recommended, and I fully support this."

ᵃ In those cases where a long-standing patient is reluctant or refuses to participate in UDT and is likely to be physically dependent on the opioid class of drug, a significant tightening of boundaries (e.g., very limited prescriptions, more frequent follow-up appointments) may serve to help manage risk, in lieu of formal participation in the UDT process.

---

is valuable in terms of long-term diabetic outcomes. We also know that the information can be valuable as a tool in motivating or maintaining changes around glycemic control, including adherence to a prescribed diet and exercise program. Finally, we do it because it has become a standard of care in diabetic management. Completing the accountability circuit, clinician adherence to these standards is increasingly and routinely judged by health systems and payers and may serve as a metric for financial reward or punishment.

Using this example as a paradigm for optimizing and aligning best practices with incentives and accountability, UDT should be introduced in a positive and open manner to staff and patients as a routine a matter, without undue emotional overlay. It should be emphasized that drug testing is performed as part of an ongoing commitment to addressing risk and preventing harm in the use of controlled substances for patients and their loved ones. Equally important, it is a tool that can be used as a stepping-off point for broader clinician–patient discussions about lifestyle issues and adherence that might otherwise be difficult to initiate.

Certainly one of the more difficult situations is with a longstanding patient whom a clinician has known for years. There is a tendency to believe that the UDT is unimportant here. In fact, while we know that drug and alcohol use varies over the life cycle, the fact is that we really only *believe* we know who in our practice is, might be, or is not using drugs problematically. Having a policy of practice-wide application can help reduce the risk of unfairly stigmatizing any one group of patients. That certainly does not imply that everyone is tested with the same degree of frequency, but it should mean that we talk with everyone about drug testing and its role in one's practice.

As a general rule, drug testing should be discussed with every patient. As well, it would be reasonable to assume that, all things considered, a drug test would be obtained, at least initially and again at a frequency that ongoing clinical judgement recommends, from all patients where controlled substances are prescribed. It should also be remembered that in those retrospective assessments of patients that ultimately become significant problems, one of the most commonly missing elements of the clinical record is the UDT result.

There are many valid pragmatic clinical reasons why a UDT sample might not be collected per usual clinic routine in certain patients, but efforts should be made to overcome impediments to urine testing for patients on chronic opioid therapy. However, if collecting a urine sample is simply too difficult, defaulting to blood sample testing may become necessary.

DEFINITIVE VERSUS QUANTITATIVE TESTING

If we are talking about definitive testing, we should be contrasting it with presumptive testing insofar as the clinician is given specific information about the presence or absence of any given analyte. Unfortunately, definitive testing and quantitative testing are often linked together, which can lead to an overreliance on the numerical values sometimes associated with these definitive tests.

As a general rule, immunoassay testing uses an antibody–antigen interaction to identify classes of drugs. Combined chromatographic/spectrometric testing such as gas chromatography (GC)/MS or LC/MS-MS are able to specifically and definitively identify many primary as well as secondary analytes. Unfortunately, this precision typically comes with the added cost of more sophisticated sample preparation and analysis.[14]

Clearly, in the typical pain practice the sole reliance on presumptive testing is with significant limitations. To know that the urine is positive for a member of the opiate class of drugs is relevant (if the patient is not supposed to be taking a member of this therapeutic class) but can be clinically misleading if the patient is being prescribed a member of this class of drug. In this case, it is not simply enough to know that they are "positive" by presumptive testing; they must be positive for the correct (e.g., prescribed) drug. This usually requires more sophisticated testing such as combined chromatographic/spectrometric testing such as LC/MS-MS.

But when we look at definitive testing, we know exactly which analyte is being reported. This is often critical information as it relates to the drug-using or drug-prescribed patient population. A currently debated question is the role of the quantitative values associated with these definitive tests.

In some cases, quantification is critical. Without it, it would be difficult to distinguish between primary analytes (i.e., drugs that are being prescribed and are being taken by the patient) compared to secondary analytes (i.e., metabolites that are likely due to the appropriate use of primary therapeutic agents rather than the concurrent use of other unprescribed therapeutic agents).

Metabolite Identification

For example, a patient being prescribed morphine may under certain circumstances be found to have hydromorphone present in the sample.[26] By simple presumptive testing, this would likely be reported as "positive" for opiates. By definitive testing, it would likely be reported as "positive morphine" and "positive hydromorphone." At this point, the clinician does not know if this patient is appropriately using the prescribed morphine or has relapsed back to a past problem with hydromorphone. Only through quantitative analysis can this question be answered. Quantitative results are most useful to the interpreting laboratory scientist, who will typically comment that the presence of hydromorphone is "likely a metabolite of morphine." Notice the word "likely." It certainly is possible that the hydromorphone could be due to the use of illicit or unprescribed hydromorphone, but if the amount is merely a fraction of the more primary morphine metabolites, it most likely is due to morphine metabolism. Of course this highlights the reason morphine is a poor choice in a patient where hydromorphone misuse is a distinct possibility (i.e., a former hydromorphone abuser; see Figure 4.1).

This point is relevant because although it is assumed that the added value of quantification of all definitive tests should be without question, unfortunately, this is not necessarily true.

Other than increased cost, the quantified information can be more dangerous in a very real clinical context. In many cases, clinicians faced with quantitative values that have increased compared to previous values interpret this as evidence of increased drug use. Conversely, where the values have diminished, that might be interpreted as evidence of dose reduction. These conclusions may be wrong, purely on the basis of technical variance. This is especially true when some laboratories are proposing that individual lab results can be compared to proprietary databases of "known compliant" patients to further add "scientific" validity to these dubious interpretations.[14]

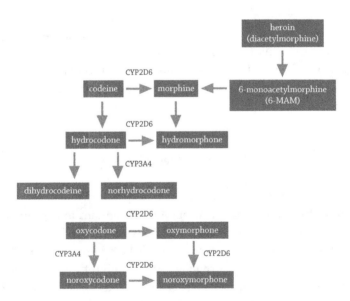

Figure 4.1. Examples of metabolism of opioids, showing major cytochrome P450 enzymes involved in phase 1 metabolism. Not comprehensive pathways but may explain the presence of apparently unprescribed drugs.
Used with permission of the authors. Gourlay D, Heit H, Caplan YH. *Urine Drug Testing in Clinical Practice—The Art and Science of Patient Care*, 6th ed. Baltimore, MD: Johns Hopkins University School of Medicine; 2015.

Drug Elimination Monitoring

So what use is the quantitative result to a busy clinician beyond distinguishing between primary and secondary analytes? In some cases, patient care may benefit from quantitative monitoring of the elimination of certain drugs from the patient. For example, say a patient who has been an acknowledged marijuana user has agreed to discontinue use of this drug as part of an agreed-upon treatment plan. In this case, steadily falling THC levels over time are supportive of treatment adherence. Equally important, an unexpected increase in the quantified value *could* represent relapse back to cannabis use—certainly it merits an open and honest discussion with the patient. Clearly, with careful thought and documentation, quantitative results can be of significant importance in clinical care. Having said this, it would be unwise to suggest that, in all cases, quantified results are either better or even necessary. Rational laboratory utilization always requires careful clinical thought before *and* after ordering a test.

ROLE OF UDT IN THE NONOPIOID-USING PATIENT POPULATION

In many respects, UDT is an underutilized clinical test. For many who use drug testing, it is largely restricted to patients who are being considered for or who are already being prescribed members of the opioid class of drug. UDT can have a much more clinically useful role in patient care.

There are many clinical scenarios where unexpected use *or nonuse* of mood-altering substances can adversely affect patient outcome. Take, as an example, the patient who struggles with anxiety. A simple urine drug test can identify the unprescribed use of benzodiazepines or chronic use of alcohol that might otherwise go undetected, especially if the patient sees the use of these agents as a means of coping with stressful situations.

Similarly, an elderly patient may find that the use of medications prescribed to her by various practitioners is information that does not need to be shared among them. Problematic drug use in this population can be very difficult to identify, especially if the patient has been using these drugs for some time without apparent harm. As we age, drug metabolism patterns can change dramatically, leading to changes in mental status that might be misinterpreted. A UDT report that rules out the presence of cognitively impairing drugs can help direct the treatment team toward other potentially treatable causes for the presenting symptom cluster.

INTERPRETATION OF UDT RESULTS

Urine drug testing has, in some practices, been used to identify "legitimate" pain patients. But the very notion of "legitimate" pain patients is clinically problematic. Certainly there are some patients who seek controlled substances either to maintain a SUD or to obtain stock for the criminal trafficking of these substances. In the former case, this is a patient who may struggle with a complex, treatable SUD. They need to be identified as such and referred to treatment for this "legitimate" illness. The latter are engaged in criminal behavior, and, as such, clinicians should do all that is reasonably in their power to interrupt their supply of drugs.

Being engaged in the criminal trafficking of controlled substances does not exclude the possibility of a treatable medical condition such as chronic pain. It does, however, present risk to the public, to the patient, and to the practitioner. In these cases, criminal activity needs to be interdicted, with the hope that appropriate medical treatment will follow.[2] In either case, the likelihood of treatment adherence without specialized and highly structured care, if at all and if indicated for a medical condition, is remote.

TREATMENT ADHERENCE

The very idea of treatment adherence means different things to different people. For some, the notion of treatment adherence is synonymous with "compliance," that is, taking exactly what the practitioner prescribed, in the amount ordered, at precise times. In reality, chronic pain requires a much broader approach to understanding treatment adherence.

For the typical chronic pain patient without a medication use problem or psychiatric condition, a capable clinician will provide the patient with guidance and limits around how many and how often certain medications should be used and advice to report problems (e.g., adverse effects) if they occur. The prescriber then expects the patient to follow these instructions, with latitude for use of breakthrough pain doses as needed to optimize pain control and function as circumstances dictate. The patient is considered to be adherent if he or she does not run out of medications early and they return for scheduled follow-up appointments as scheduled.

Closer scrutiny of adherence behavior in a wide variety of conditions suggests that a range of behaviors is actually occurring among "typical" patients. The concept of "average" use over a one-month period allows for a lot of daily variability before the trigger of "running out early" is met. "Borrowing from tomorrow to pay for today"[27] is a concept that many struggling pain patients can relate to in terms of using "enough" medication to get through a difficult time, "hoping" that the times ahead are going to be easier and so require less medication. Asking as simple a question as "What's the most medication you have had to use in a 24-hour period?" can be much more illuminating than simply looking for patterns of running out of medications early.

UDT is actually severely limited in terms of what it can and cannot tell about how medication is used on a daily basis. These limitations should not be considered fatal flaws. To a certain extent, the UDT is intended to help basically well-intended patients people make healthy choices and possibly prevent potential catastrophes. The UDT remains one of the few scientifically objective tools to assess drug use (both prescription and otherwise) in a patient population we know will not always be able to make good decisions. But it is critical to remember—we cannot use UDT to count pills.

Behavioral Elements of UDT

There is a temptation to focus on the analytical aspects of UDT, even though we have acknowledged that its use in assessing treatment adherence is somewhat limited. There is, however, another dimension to the clinical use of UDT in patient care. This dimension might best be considered in terms of behavioral indicators.

For example, a patient might have readily agreed to participate in UDT "in theory" but when actually asked to provide a sample may express doubts about the appropriateness of the request. This provide a subtle clue as to what may or may not be found in the UDT specimen. Similarly, some patients will agree to provide a sample but ultimately "never get around" to providing one. Again, this should alert the clinician to the opportunity to have a full and frank discussion with the patient about the reasons behind these behaviors, tightening prescription boundaries accordingly.

It is not uncommon for clinicians to be confronted with information (including laboratory test results) that alone offers no definitive answer. As an example, consider the sample that is positive for the cocaine metabolite, benzoylecgonine. In some cases, the patient may simply acknowledge the result as correct: "I made a bad choice at a party on the weekend." Arguably, if the patient is asking for help with a potential drug problem, he or she can be treated much more compassionately than one who expresses a fundamental belief in his or her *right* to periodically use cocaine—even while being prescribed controlled substances—defying the trust that had been promised. In the former case, referral for assessment of a potential SUD is appropriate, while significantly tightening the boundaries around treatment with controlled substances. Interval dispensing,[28] more frequent contact with counselors, and more frequent visits with random UDT, to mention a few strategies, can all be thought of as defensible, rational, and compassionate clinical care.[28]

The patient who breaks a promise and exerts her or his "right" to use cocaine should be addressed in an entirely different manner that does not include continued prescription of controlled substances. This patient has openly acknowledged a unwillingness to adhere to what had been a mutually agreed-upon treatment plan. But what if the circumstances are not so crisply defined?

Consider the individual who presents with an abnormal UDT result (e.g., benzoylecgonine positive, prescribed opioid negative) with no apparent explanation. The laboratory verifies the test results: there is no doubt of the results, but why and what to do about it?

The practitioner may be tempted to confront the patient with this information in an accusatory way that will invariably lead to defensiveness, shame, and a sense of imminent threat (abandonment) on the part of the patient. The result is a fractured therapeutic relationship and likely termination of the relationship. There must be a better way to handle these sorts of cases.

A defensible and rational approach would be to simply accept the patient's story as offered *but* to restate the fact that this result is unacceptable, for whatever the reason might be. As such, the problem can be addressed by a significant tightening of the boundaries around use of controlled substances. It may also be appropriate to refer the patient for more definitive investigation/consultation to rule out a SUD. As stated before, the only truly incorrect response is to do nothing. Ultimately, abnormal or unexpected results must not be ignored. Adherence can only be improved by strengthening therapeutic bonds. For many, this can be a long and arduous road, not unlike the work of managing brittle diabetes in the face of severe dietary indiscretion.

To many patients, the science of UDT is a mystery. While more information now exists on the Internet on how to manipulate UDT, most patients are not this sophisticated. In this regard, there is sometimes a fear that UDT will reveal much more to the prescriber than it is actually able to do. This uncertainty, when coupled with open-ended questions by the practitioner in discussing the patient's behavior, can sometimes produce information that would not otherwise be revealed. When used to enhance clinical care, we refer to this as "patient-centered UDT"; when used to deny care, we see this as an abuse of a valuable clinical tool.

MISLEADING TEST RESULTS

As a scientific tool, UDT can only tell us what is detected and what is not detected in terms of analytes tested for. It is a common misconception that drug testing tests for "all drugs." While the methods currently used are very good, certain drugs and drug classes may require sample preparation that is only available on specific request. For example, the potent analgesic fentanyl may be present in such small quantities that its detection, even when specifically requested, can be difficult. On the other hand, the primary metabolite nor-fentanyl is often present in larger quantities and so may be easier to detect.

False Negative/False Positive Results

One of the more problematic uses of UDT is the absolute determination of treatment compliance through the detection of the prescribed medication and/or its metabolite. It is not always the case that if the patient actually took the drug the lab test will always report it as detected. A host of factors can create this "false negative" result, suggestive of poor adherence. This finding needs to be corroborated before conclusions are drawn.[3,14,29,30]

There is another area where UDT results can be misleading, and that is when aberrant behavior is hidden within seemingly "expected" UDT results. The one drug that a person can abuse with impunity is the one a clinician would expect to find in his or her urine.

For example, a patient who has been prescribed a morphine-based analgesic may supplement his or her use with medications obtained by doctor-shopping, overuse of medication stockpiles that they have stored up over time, or even illicitly obtained drugs (either morphine itself or heroin that is metabolized to morphine). Contrary to claims made by several laboratories, quantitative analysis of urine will not yield reliable information about patterns of drug use. The only way to address this is through a combination of laboratory and clinical evaluation. Patients who are clinically stable are likely to be using their medications appropriately—if they are not, it is unlikely that they will remain clinically stable for long.

On the other hand, the choice of medication prescribed to a patient with a past history of drug abuse can help increase the sensitivity of laboratory results tremendously. For example, a morphine-based analgesic would be a poor choice in a former heroin user. Since the only thing that distinguishes appropriate prescription morphine use from illicit heroin relapse is a very short-lived intermediary called mono-acetyl morphine (6-MAM),

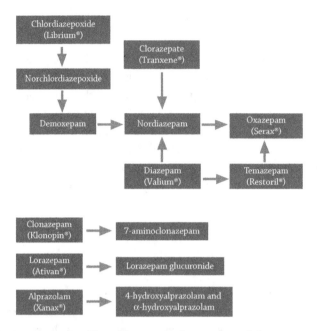

Figure 4.2. Some examples of benzodiazepine pathways of metabolism.
Used with permission of the authors. Gourlay D, Heit H, Caplan YH. *Urine Drug Testing in Clinical Practice—The Art and Science of Patient Care*, 6th ed. Baltimore, MD: Johns Hopkins University School of Medicine; 2015.

the expected observation of morphine in the urine would make early detection of heroin relapse virtually impossible. The avoidance of morphine or drugs that include morphine in their metabolic pathway is recommended (Figure 4.1).

In a similar fashion, it is important to remember that the metabolic pathways for certain classes of drugs are complex, often producing intermediaries that are, in themselves, commonly prescribed medication, that can then lead to ambiguities in interpretation of lab results. An example of the complexities of interpreting UDT test results employing the pathways of metabolism fro benzodiazepines is illustrated in figure 4.2.

PATIENT-CENTERED RESPONSES TO ANOMALOUS RESULTS

The reflex reaction for many clinicians faced with abnormal UDT results is to fire the patient.[29] In the author's opinion, this is not only unwise; it is largely unnecessary. There are a multitude of more therapeutically beneficial (health-promoting) approaches to the question of how to address abnormal UDT results. There really is only one absolutely "wrong" approach, and that is to do nothing. Ignoring UDT data only lets the patient down, in terms of missing a potential opportunity to interrupt a downward spiral into active drug abuse and addiction. It also fails to address the moral responsibility we have as prescribers to help prevent potentially dangerous drugs from being diverted into the community from legitimate medical channels.

USE OF ALTERNATIVE TEST MATRICES IN CLINICAL TESTING

Over the past few years, the choice of test matrix for clinical testing has largely remained with urine. As a sample, urine has been described as the nearly perfect test matrix. It is simple to collect and store, cheap to prepare and analyze, and is minimally invasive (painless, no medical risk) in terms of intruding into the donor's life to collect the samples. As well, the windows of detection for most commonly tested substances falls within a two- to three-day range (Table 4.4). Of course there are other matrixes to test. Hair, saliva, sweat, breath and blood are all valid samples for drug testing, depending on the reason(s) for ordering the test and what question(s) are being asked[31] (see Figure 4.3).

Table 4.4. APPROXIMATE WINDOWS OF DETECTION OF DRUG IN URINE

General Detection	Drug Time in Urine[a]
Amphetamines	Up to 3 days
THCA (depending on the grade and frequency of marijuana use)	
– Single use	– 1 to 3 days
– Chronic use	– Up to 30 days
Cocaine	Hours
– Benzoylecgonine after cocaine use	– 2 to 4 days
Opiates (morphine, codeine)	2 to 3 days
– Heroin (diacetylmorphine)	– 3 to 5 minutes
– 6-MAM	– 25 to 30 minutes
Methadone	Up to 3 days
– EDDP (methadone metabolite)	– Up to 6 days
Benzodiazepines (depending on the specific agent and quantity used)	Days to weeks

---

Note: 6-MAM = 6-monoacetylmorphine; EDDP = 2-ethylidene-1,5-dimethyl-3,3-diphenylpyrrolidine; THCA = delta-9-tetrahydrocannabinol-9-carboxylic acid.
[a] The detection time of drugs formulated into extended-release or transdermal dosage formulations may be longer.

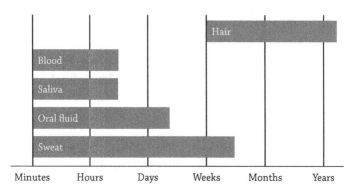

Figure 4.3. Relative detection times of drugs in biologic specimens. Note: Apparently over-lapping detection times will not necessarily yield matching positive or negative results in all the alternate matrices.

Used with permission of the authors. Gourlay D, Heit H, Caplan YH. Urine Drug Testing in Clinical Practice—The Art and Science of Patient Care. 6th ed. 2015, Baltimore, MD: Johns Hopkins University School of Medicine.

CONCLUSIONS

Although the use of UDT has become something of a de facto standard of care in the treatment of patients with chronic pain prescribed controlled substances, it has been elevated to this level in the absence of any scientific evidence to support this standard. In fact, Starrels et al.[11] in their review of treatment agreements and drug testing commented on the lack of uniformity in application of drug testing in clinical care, making comparisons with articles dealing with UDT difficult.

To a certain extent, UDT has become such a rapidly accepted, albeit controversial, part of clinical care because of the significant prescription drug problem that has evolved over the past decade. This makes the proper interpretation of these tests all the more important. At this time, we believe that there is a need to ensure that the use of UDT remains within the context of truly patient-centered care and the broader construct of adherence. To do otherwise runs a significant risk of our violating the very first rule of medicine: *primum non nocere*.

UDT as it pertains to enhancing treatment adherence is more about engaging the patient in an often challenging clinical dialogue rather than ensuring that some arbitrary set of processes of care are met and enforced. Medicine is by necessity a profession of making difficult decisions with incomplete information. While we are making great strides forward in the science of drug testing, we must respect the significant limitations imposed on us by our art.

REFERENCES

1. Lipman, AG. The controversy over urine drug testing in pain management patient monitoring. *J Pain Palliat Care Pharmacother.* 2013;27(4):320–321.

2. Gourlay DL. Heit H, Almarhezi A. Universal precautions in pain medicine: a rational approach to the management of chronic pain. *Pain Med.* 2005;6(2):107–112.

3. Heit HA, Gourlay DL. Using urine drug testing to support healthy boundaries in clinical care. *J Opioid Manag.* 2015;11(1):7–12.

4. Buchman DZ, Ho A, Illes J. You present like a drug addict: patient and clinician perspectives on trust and trustworthiness in chronic pain management. *Pain Med.* 2016;17(8):1394–13406.

5. Reisfield GM, Maschke K. Urine drug testing in long-term opioid therapy: ethical considerations. *Clin J Pain.* 2014;30(8):679–684.

6. Krishnamurthy P, Ranganathan G, Williams C, Doulatram G. Impact of urine drug screening on no shows and dropouts among chronic pain patients: a propensity-matched cohort study. *Pain Physician.* 2016;19 (2):89–100.

7. Garg RK, Fulton-Kehoe D, Turner JA, et al. Changes in opioid prescribing for Washington workers' compensation claimants after implementation of an opioid dosing guideline for chronic noncancer pain: 2004 to 2010. *J Pain.* 2013;14(12):1620–1628.

8. Nuckols TK, Anderson L, Popescu I, et al. Opioid prescribing: a systematic review and critical appraisal of guidelines for chronic pain. *Ann Intern Med.* 2014;160(1):38–47.

9. Von Korff M, Dublin S, Walker RL, et al. The impact of opioid risk reduction initiatives on high-dose opioid prescribing for patients on chronic opioid therapy. *J Pain.* 2016;17(1):101–110.

10. Alford DP. Opioid prescribing for chronic pain—Achieving the right balance through education. *N Engl J Med.* 2016;374(4):301–303.

11. Starrels JL, Becker WC, Alford DP, Kapoor A, Williams AR, Turner BJ. Systematic review: treatment agreements and urine drug testing to reduce opioid misuse in patients with chronic pain. *Ann Intern Med.* 2010;152(11):712–720.

12. Heit HA, Gourlay DL. Tackling the difficult problem of prescription opioid misuse. *Ann Intern Med.* 2010;152(11):747–748.

13. Federation of State Medical Boards. *Model Policy on the Appropriate Use of Opioid Analgesics in the Treatment of Pain.* Euless, TX: Federation of State Medical Boards; 2013.

14. Gourlay D, Heit H, Caplan YH. *Urine Drug Testing in Clinical Practice—The Art and Science of Patient Care,* 6th ed. Baltimore, MD: Johns Hopkins University School of Medicine; 2015.

15. Heit HA, Gourlay DL. Urine drug testing in pain medicine. *J Pain Symptom Manage.* 2004;27(3):260–267.

16. Connell PH. Urine testing for the presence of drugs in the treatment of drug dependent persons with special reference to inpatient treatment. *Int Pharmacopsychiatry.* 1972;7(1–4):199–204.

17. Weaver C. Doctors cash in on drug tests for seniors and Medicare pays the bill. *Wall Street Journal.* Nov. 10, 2014.

18. Hendee WR, Becker GJ, Borgstede JP, et al. Addressing overutilization in medical imaging. *Radiology.* 2010;257(1):240–245.

19. Reisfield GM, Goldberger BA, Bertholf RL. Choosing the right laboratory: a review of clinical and forensic toxicology services for urine drug testing in pain management. *J Opioid Manag.* 2015;11(1):37–44.

20. Katz N, Fanciullo G. Role of urine toxicology testing in the management of chronic opioid therapy. *Clin J Pain.* 2002;18(4 Suppl.):S76–S82.

21. Markman JD, Barbosa WA, Gewandter JS, et al. Interpretation of urine drug testing results in patients using transdermal buprenorphine preparations for the treatment of chronic noncancer pain. *Pain Med.* 2015;16(6):1132–1136.

22. Shults T. *The Medical Review Officer Handbook,* 10th ed. Research Triangle Park, NC: Quadrangle Research; 2014.

23. Kirsh KL, Heit HA, Huskey A, Strickland J, Egan K, Passik SD. Trends in drug use from urine drug testing of addiction treatment clients. *J Opioid Manag.* 2015;11(1):61–68.

24. Gourlay D, Heit H. Universal precautions: a matter of mutual trust and responsibility. *Pain Med.* 2006;7(2):210–211; author reply 212.

25. Fishman SM. Trust and pharmaco-vigilance in pain medicine. *Pain Med.* 2005;6(5):392; discussion 396.

26. Cone EJ, Heit HA, Caplan YH, Gourlay D. Evidence of morphine metabolism to hydromorphone in pain patients chronically treated with morphine. *J Anal Toxicol.* 2006;30(1):1–5.

27. Heit HA, Gourlay D. Treatment of chronic pain in patients with a history of substance abuse. In: Balantyne JC, Fishman SM, Rathmell JP, eds. *Bonica's Management of Pain.* Philadelphia: Lippincott, Williams and Wilkins; 2010.

28. Gourlay D, Heit HA. Universal precautions revisited: managing the inherited pain patient. *Pain Med.* 2009;10(Suppl 2):S115–123.

29. Gourlay D. Compliance monitoring in chronic pain management. In: Balantyne JC, Fishman SM, Rathmell JP, ed. *Bonica's Management of Pain.* Philadelphia: Lippicott, Williams and Wilkins; 2010.

30. Heit HA, Gourlay D. Urine drug testing in pain medicine. *J Pain Symptom Manage.* 2004;27(3):260–267.

31. Caplan YH, Goldberger A. Alternative specimens for workplace drug testing. *J Anal Toxicol.* 2001;25(5):396–399.

CHAPTER 5

ↄ\ɔ

Adherence to Weight Loss and Physical Activity

E. AMY JANKE AND DAVID E. GOODRICH

INTRODUCTION

Weight management and regular physical activity each contribute to health generally and have specific benefits for the individual with pain. Adults who maintain a healthy weight and remain active and physically fit are less likely to develop chronic pain, or if they suffer from chronic pain it may be more manageable. For patients with chronic pain, those who manage their weight and maintain both daily activity levels and regular exercise are more likely to have favorable pain intensity, pain disability, and quality of life outcomes compared to those who have heavier weights and/or are inactive. Physical activity contributes to improved health in many areas beyond weight management. However, given that inactivity is a risk factor for obesity, regular physical activity is a particularly powerful approach to improving health and a component of evidence-based approaches to achieve weight loss.

Obesity is a high-prevalence condition associated with significant morbidity, increased mortality, and economic cost. Given its wide-reaching negative health impact and resistance to intervention, obesity should be a concern addressed by all healthcare providers (HCP). Despite efforts to promote prevention and achieve sustained weight loss, obesity continues to be a global public health crisis. Rates of obesity are increasing worldwide, with prevalence rates at or exceeding 50% in some countries.[1] In 2010, 35% of the US adult population was obese,[2] and more than two-thirds of US adults are either overweight, obese, or extremely obese.[2] Obesity-related conditions include leading causes of preventable death,[3,4] and annual US obesity-attributable medical expenditures are staggering and estimated at $147 billion, with $34 billion financed by Medicare and $28 billion financed by Medicaid.[5]

Overweight and obesity are defined most commonly according to body mass index (BMI). Overweight is defined as a BMI of 25 kg/m^2 to 29.9 kg/m^2 and obesity as a BMI of $\geq$30 kg/m^2, cut points that are associated with increased risk for morbidity and mortality compared to individuals with a BMI in the normal range (BMI 18.5 to <25.0 kg/m^2).[6] Physical inactivity and poor diet are among the chief risk factors for obesity.[7] Accordingly, current treatment guidelines for obesity recommend comprehensive and intensive lifestyle interventions that include dietary modification, physical activity, and behavioral strategies.[6]

RELATIONSHIP BETWEEN WEIGHT AND PAIN

Chronic pain and obesity are increasingly recognized as a common and troubling comorbidity. Individuals with persistent pain and who are overweight or obese are likely to experience increased disability, poorer psychosocial function, reduced quality of life, attenuated treatment responsiveness, and increased healthcare utilization and cost.[8] Increased weight is a risk factor for poor pain outcomes and several pain-related conditions, making adherence to weight loss an important treatment target with high relevance to pain as well as overall health.

There appears to be linear, incremental relationship between BMI and pain report such that as BMI increases risk for pain complaints also increases.[9] A recent telephone survey of 1 million adults demonstrated convincingly that individuals with higher BMIs are more prone to experiencing daily pain, an association that remains significant even after controlling for type of pain conditions, gender, and age.[9] Specifically, compared to individuals with BMIs at or below 25, 20% more pain was reported by those who had a BMI 25 to 29.9 (overweight), 68% more pain for those with BMIs 30 to 34.9 (obese I), 136% more pain for those with BMIs 35 to 39.9 (obese II), and 254% more pain for those with BMIs $\geq$ 40 (obese III).[9]

Most remarkable is the variety in pain conditions shown to be associated with obesity. In one community-based twin study, compared to normal-weight twins, those with a BMI $\geq$ 25 were more likely to report physician-diagnosed low back pain, tension-type or migraine headache, fibromyalgia, abdominal pain, and chronic widespread pain.[10] Longitudinal studies and meta-analytic designs have demonstrated that the presence of being overweight and obese increases the risk for back pain over time,[11] and similar findings have been demonstrated for osteoarthritis of the knee,[12] hip,[13] and hand.[14] Rates of obesity in fibromyalgia have been shown to be high, ranging from ranging from 47% to 73%,[15,16] and overweight individuals may be at 60% to 80% greater risk for developing fibromyalgia[17] with increasing weight associated with rising symptom severity and disability.[18] Obese individuals are at greater risk of having headaches generally, and specifically obesity appears to increase the risk of migraine by an estimated 40% to 80%, a risk that increases with higher levels of BMI.[19]

Pathways linking excessive weight to specific pain conditions are likely complex and vary depending on the nature of the comorbidity. For some conditions, such as osteoarthritis of the knee, mechanical and structural changes may be among the critical risk factors.[20] For others such as migraine, inflammatory and metabolic factors may play a larger role.[21] Behavioral and psychosocial factors are often cited as a common risk factor for both pain and weight and likely mechanisms that may either initiate and/or maintain a relationship between the two conditions.

Encouragingly, weight loss is generally associated with improvement in pain symptoms[22] and may prevent or delay the onset of conditions such as osteoarthritis.[23] Both lifestyle interventions and bariatric surgery appear to have a positive impact on pain symptoms for individuals with osteoarthritis,[24] fibromyalgia,[25] and headache,[21] among other conditions. While much remains unknown about targeting weight loss in individuals with specific pain conditions, it appears lifestyle treatments that target both dietary change and physical activity are promising to achieve both weight loss and improved pain outcomes.[26] Weight loss strategies—such as physical activity, contingency management, and coping strategies—often overlap with behavioral approaches included in psychological programs for pain.[27] Such findings suggest that adherence to these approaches may be a powerful and synergistic method to address both pain and weight concerns as well as improving overall morbidity and mortality in this population, particularly given the increased risk for pain and disability associated with higher levels of BMI.

While weight loss is associated with multiple health benefits, including pain reduction, it is challenging to achieve sustained weight loss in most clinical environments. Perceived barriers to weight loss are often high, and patient adherence to lifestyle change can be low. Patients and their HCPs report pain is a barrier to weight loss and increased weight is a barrier to chronic pain self-management.[28,29] Evidence from patients enrolled in treatments focused solely on weight loss or pain self-management management support this—patients with comorbid pain and weight concerns experience poorer weight loss[30] and pain management[31] outcomes in interventions with a singular disease focus.

A number of barriers to weight loss face the patient with persistent pain, including low self-efficacy for physical activity due to pain and altered eating behavior in response to pain.[32] However, evidence suggests that motivation to maintain lifestyle changes that contribute to weight loss may be the biggest hurdle facing patients with pain.[29] Motivation is an important predictor of weight loss success[33] and viewed theoretically as an important precursor to behavioral change broadly for patients with pain[34] and specifically important to treatment adherence for weight loss.[35] Accordingly, weight loss interventions for individuals with pain should address patient motivation as one approach to increase adherence.

ADHERENCE AND WEIGHT LOSS FOR INDIVIDUALS WITH PAIN: A CONCEPTUAL MODEL
Defining Adherence

There is a strong association between treatment adherence and weight loss. In clinical trials comparing behavioral approaches for weight loss, adherence is defined as the extent to which participants remained engaged in the weight loss program and met specific program goals or recommended clinical guidelines for diet and/or physical activity. In these clinical trials, adherence was most strongly associated with weight loss and improvements in disease-related outcomes.[36–38] Despite many commercial options available to achieve weight loss, no one approach has proven to be better than another—the best diet for the individual patient is the one he or she is most likely adhere to.

Unfortunately, achieving significant weight loss is a challenge, and weight re-gain is common. Adherence to lifestyle changes is key to sustained benefits associated with healthy diet and physical activity,[39] yet change can occur slowly, and the majority of individuals do not maintain behavioral changes and/or weight loss over time. Across behavioral and pharmacological interventions, typically only moderate weight loss is achieved via treatments that include reduced-energy diet, physical activity, and/or pharmacological intervention, and this weight loss typically begins to plateau at 6 months and stabilize at 12 months.[40]

When weight loss (and maintenance of weight loss) is the primary goal against which adherence is measured, unfortunately the evidence suggests that improvements are modest and difficult to maintain. Both patient and HCP may feel frustrated and demoralized when, despite best efforts, little weight loss is achieved. This may be particularly true in the case of achieving weight loss in the patient with pain. An important consideration for adherence related to either weight loss or physical activity in those with pain is understanding the patient's unique concerns and challenges. Unreasonable expectations on the part of the patient and HCP must be tempered. Just as patients often present in treatment with expectations of fast pain relief with minimal lifestyle change,[41] so too do they have high expectations for significant weight loss in a brief period of time.[42] Conversely, HCPs often have negative or stereotypical views of patients with higher BMIs, viewing them as unlikely to succeed in achieving meaningful weight loss.[43]

Rather than adhering to unrealistic and inappropriate expectations, adherence must be defined according to guidelines for weight loss and physical activity, current evidence about appropriate trajectories of change and maintenance in this population, and patient-driven, mutually agreed-upon goals. While traditionally viewed in treatment as a binary outcome, adherence for the behavioral changes required for weight loss is a complex process influenced by multiple factors across time. Although the focus of this chapter is on the individual patient and HCP, the process of adherence is also influenced by the systems and communities within which it occurs.[44] These environmental factors significantly influence outcomes, and while many of these are beyond the scope of the current discussion, all of the concerns and recommendations discussed here at the patient and-HCP level are also influenced by this larger context.

HCPs should focus on increasing adherence to the healthy behaviors often associated with weight loss, including a proper diet and consistently engaging in physical activity. Despite the likelihood that sustained weight loss is unlikely and that weight tends to increase with age, evidence shows that weight loss of 5% from baseline can have a positive impact on morbidity and mortality.[6] Even maintaining one's weight may be an appropriate goal with corresponding health benefits. The behaviors associated with weight loss can positively impact multiple domains even in the absence of significant weight loss. Physical fitness and increased physical activity can reduce obesity-related health risks in individuals with high BMI without weight loss.[45] A patient-centered, evidence-based practice approach to identifying and prioritizing goals and strategies will promote achieving lasting behavior change. Goals and associated intervention strategies should be based upon current guidelines and evidence in the field, patient needs and preferences, and consideration of socioecological factors demonstrated to influence adherence and patient motivation.

A Socioecological Model of Adherence

Patient Motivation and Adherence

A cornerstone of adherence is patient motivation; without it, successful engagement with any self-management behaviors—including those associated with weight loss and physical activity—remains unlikely. For self-management to be effective, patients must identify, engage, evaluate, and maintain a number of behavior changes over time. Because motivation to engage in this process of change is an important precursor to a successful outcome, the role of motivation in behavior change has been either explicitly identified or implied by numerous models of health behavior change. A synthesis of these models by Jensen and colleagues[34] has led to the creation of a general model of motivation for pain self-management that is particularly useful when considering the needs of the patient with pain (Figure 5.1).

Motivational models have as a primary end point patient behavior change that increases health, promotes function, and engages the patient in the treatment process. Importantly, these models also describe the relationship between motivation and behavior change as a process. Motivation is not a fixed state or a stable trait; rather, it is fluid and open to influence. In their motivational model of pain, Jensen and colleagues distill factors that influence one's motivation or "readiness to change" as being either (a) beliefs about the importance of a particular behavior or (b) self-efficacy about one's ability to engage in the behavior.[34] One may be described as more or less ready to change—and thus more or less likely to engage in a particular behavior—depending on his or her beliefs about that behavior. The model describes the relationship between important constructs in motivation and adherence—self-efficacy, perceived importance, and readiness to change—and the relationships among these and has empirical support.[46]

While existing models of health behavior change—including the motivational model of pain self-management—provide useful conceptual frameworks to understand adherence, they are limited in that they typically focus primarily on individual beliefs and behaviors. While individual factors such as these are shown to influence weight loss and physical activity, other factors significantly influence motivation and adherence to these goals. Given

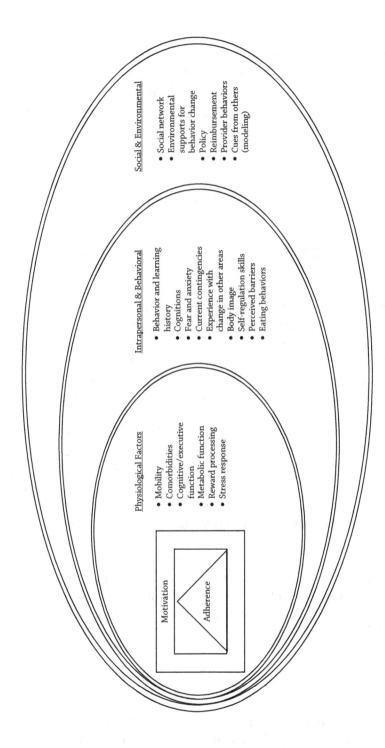

Figure 5.1. Socioecological model of adherence.

the definition of adherence as a complex behavioral process influenced by multiple factors, including the systems and communities in which it occurs, a socioecological model of adherence provides a framework to understand weight loss and physical activity in the patient with persistent pain. This model describes the relationship between adherence and motivation as influenced by a number of factors interacting across three broad domains: the physiological, intrapersonal and behavioral, and social environmental. Thus behavioral adherence is the result of the unique, dynamic interactions that occur across these domains for each individual patient.

Physiological Domain

While weight loss is an outcome that is highly influenced by patient behavior, too many HCPs conceptualize it as a behavior that is entirely at the discretion of an individual patient choice. An individual chooses what to eat (or not eat) and whether to exercise; and when they do not make the "right" choices they experience weight gain. Certainly patient behavior is one important factor, but behavior occurs within a context that includes the physiological parameters and limits unique to each individual. To suggest weight loss is entirely and completely within the explicit, rational control of the patient does not reflect what is known about weight loss/gain and reinforces already existing prejudices that obese patients are lazy and prone to failure.

There are many physiological processes that likely influence motivation for and adherence to weight loss and physical activity, either directly or indirectly. These may include the patient's mobility, metabolic function, presence of comorbidities, cognitive function, reward processing, and stress response. Each of these areas may or may not be malleable to change given the appropriate intervention, but each provides an important context of understanding the potential for adherence. Prescriptions for change frequently fail to address, or at least understand, very real limitations imposed by these physiological states. While many factors may influence adherence, sensitivity to rewards and neurocognitive deficits as new areas of investigation relevant to adherence and outcome in weight loss and health behavior change.

Sensitivity to reward

Our reward system plays an important role in our behavioral goal orientation and prioritizing. Food is a natural reward, and the food we find most rewarding is often the least healthy and most likely to contribute to weight gain. Foods that are highly palatable, widely available, and calorically dense and low in micronutrients can be especially rewarding. Behavioral responses to food and other rewards in our environment are modulated by dopamine pathways in the brain's reward centers. The consumption of fats and sugars—in particular their overconsumption—causes the release of dopamine and a state many have compared similar to drug addiction.[47]

Not everyone responds to rewards in the same way—some individuals are more sensitive to rewards and their effects than others, and those with obesity and persistent pain may be particularly sensitive to rewards. Individuals with obesity demonstrate increased food reward responsiveness and impairments in dopaminergic pathways that regulate systems with reward sensitivity.[48] The process of dieting may even further increase the reward value of food.[49] Chronic pain is a disorder that may be characterized in part by dysregulation in dopamine system function.[50] Evidence suggests that individuals in pain have a higher drive for desired rewards than those not in pain.[51] While to date there is little research examining reward drive in those with comorbid pain and obesity, there is compelling evidence from research in each area alone that some individuals with this comorbidity may experience a biological predisposition toward consumption of high-calorie foods that may present a challenge to weight management.

In order to be successful with weight loss, one typically must be able to resist the urge to eat. Yet for the patient with pain and obesity this may in fact be doubly challenging, given the inherent reward value of food. Individuals with chronic pain and obesity may be particularly vulnerable to the reinforcing effects of food reward as a means to cope with or distract them from their pain experience.[32] While there are not yet interventions that specifically address the inherent reward value of food, behavior change and weight loss have been demonstrated to reverse reward system sensitivity. Behavioral interventions may help reduce the reward value of high-calorie food items by reversing the hyperactivation of this system for calorically dense foods versus low-calorie "healthy" foods.[52] And changes in gut anatomy and/or physiology that occur secondary to gastric bypass surgery appear to positively impact hedonic food responses, suggesting an important relationship between neuronal reward circuits and gut function.[53]

Neurocognitive deficits

Both chronic pain and obesity are conditions know to be associated with neurocognitive impairment. Elevated BMI is independently associated with reduced cognitive performance across the lifespan and, in particular, deficits in executive function.[54] While the specific mechanism remains poorly understood, there is likely a bidirectional relationship between obesity and cognition. Cognitive dysfunction predicts eventual increases in BMI,[55,56] and cognitive deficits contribute to low fruit and vegetable intake and physical inactivity[57] and may mediate the reward value of food.[58] Obesity may further exacerbate pre-existing cognitive dysfunction, contributing to obesity-related cognitive decline.[59] Chronic pain appears to result in changes to both the structure and function of the brain.[60] Individuals with chronic pain demonstrate cognitive impairments across a number of domains, in particular attention and executive function[61] and working memory.[62] Unfortunately, certain treatment approaches to manage pain, such as the use of certain analgesic medications, may further augment these deficits.[61]

Cognitive deficits are problematic for adherence in a number of chronic medical conditions, and impairment has been shown to be associated with reduced medication adherence[63] and poor self-management.[64] For individuals with obesity, cognitive function is a predictor of long-term weight loss after bariatric surgery[65,66]; those with poorer cognitive function lose less weight. Cognitive function may moderate adherence following surgery in this population,[67] such that individuals with poorer function experience difficulty adhering to postsurgical recommendations that enhance weight loss.

Though neurocognitive deficits likely influence adherence outcomes, at this time there is no obvious treatment approach to address cognitive deficits for those with pain and/or weight concerns. It is unclear whether cognitive deficits observed in obesity or chronic pain would improve with treatment. However, these deficits clearly represent an important context for understanding adherence. Patients who demonstrate lower cognitive function—particularly in the domain of executive functioning—will likely struggle with the many important decisions and the behavioral changes required for a successful weight loss and/or physical activity program. These may be individuals who require additional support in the form of tools and techniques to enhance weight loss outcomes and engagement in physical activity. Of note, though untested in the area of weight and pain, cognitive remediation has been successful to address deficits associated with other medical disorders and improve adherence.[68]

Intrapersonal and Behavioral Domain

A wealth of literature demonstrates that an individual's thoughts, behaviors, and intrapersonal processes influence his or her adherence to weight loss and physical activity. There are a number of intrapersonal concepts drawn from theories/models of behavior change relevant in this domain— these include perceived barriers, self-regulation skills, body image, eating behavior, learning history, and current contingencies—and each may provide targets for intervention to achieve sustained behavior change and improved health and quality of life. Here we focus on concepts most often applied in the literature on pain, weight, and/or activity and most likely to be of relevance in understanding and addressing weight loss and physical activity in the person with pain.

Operant conditioning and behavioral economics

Weight control and sustained engagement in physical activity involve a number of behavioral decisions that take place over a sustained period of time. Operant conditioning describes the relationship between behavior and the environment: rewards increase the likelihood of a behavior reoccurring; negative consequences (punishments) decrease the likelihood.[69] Weight tends to change slowly. Many of the decisions that influence weight do not have an immediate, observable, and rewarding outcome. Indeed, long-term outcomes may be the inverse of short-term outcomes, and the relationship between eating and weight is a good example of this paradox.

Eating is an extremely rewarding activity for most individuals, particularly when it involves the consumption of palatable, high-calorie food. Yet, for an individual attempting weight loss, the momentary reward they receive from eating a high-calorie food is often inconsistent with their eventual goal of weight loss. For those attempting weight loss, immediate consequences (such as the reinforcing power of food) have more influence than the delayed negative consequence of weight gain. Behaviors are most easily established when they are rewarded immediately and often, and once established are best maintained with inconsistent, infrequent rewards. What is needed for success is the ability to delay gratification and manage temptations. To date, treatments that encourage such decision-making and provide alternative approaches to temptation management are being developed but have not yet been widely disseminated into practice.[70]

Behavioral economic theory also describes how incentives—gains and rewards, risk and loss—can influence weight loss and physical activity.[71,72] The current food environment is characterized by widely available, calorically dense yet nutrient-poor foods that are heavily marketed, inexpensive, overportioned, and confusingly labeled.[73] Given these conditions, it is very easy to make unhealthy choices even when these choices are inconsistent with one's long-term goals for weight management.[74] Indeed, not only are individuals biased toward rewards received in the moment relative to any future outcomes or rewards; they are also likely to be overly optimistic about their ability to "do better" in the future when they make poor choices.[75] Thus we are more likely to make poor choices in the present time and also believe (incorrectly) we will do better later on to compensate for the poor choice.

Behavioral economic theory has pointed to many aspects of human behavior that challenge adherence to weight loss and physical activity. Change is hard—we have a "status quo bias" and are most typically guided in our choices by what we have always done, what is easy, and what is convenient. Our activity and food habits are likely to be automated and mindless, and unfortunately these default choices tend to be unhealthy ones.[76] Our estimates about portion size and judgments about what to eat are frequently biased by external cues that distract from the true value, a concept referred to as "anchoring." For example, how much we eat has been shown to be influenced by the size of our plate or bowl and the size of the package containing our food.[76] This inherent bias can make accurate portion size estimates challenging. Weight loss is often contingent on adherence to strict controls on caloric intake, a goal that becomes nearly impossible if one cannot accurately determine calories in a portion or accurate portion size.

Behaviors are not isolated events: one behavior affects another. We often compensate for the consequences of one behavior by changing another behavior. We also are likely to substitute one unhealthy behavior for another. These processes of compensation and substitution influence adherence to weight loss and physical activity. People who begin an exercise program may find they compensate and "reward" themselves for exercising by consuming more calories. Another may decide to eat healthier by giving up fats, only to substitute high-carbohydrate foods that cause them to increase their caloric intake (rather than decrease it).[72]

Interventions based on behavioral economic theory have had some success to date. However, because they are designed to influence one's decision, either by changing the "default" settings in our environment for us or by actively offering an incentive to change behavior (such as money), they can be controversial. Contingency contracts, where individuals agree to receive certain rewards if they achieve their weight loss or physical activity goal or abide by predetermined penalties if they fail to reach their goal, have some empirical support.[77] Group insurance plans often offer rewards as part of their wellness programs, and financial incentives have been used successfully to help motivate behaviors associated with weight management, including dietary change[78] and physical activity.[79]

Self-efficacy

Self-efficacy is an important mechanism responsible for long-term, success-ful adherence to weight loss and physical activity. Self-efficacy is a belief in one's ability to perform a behavior, or set of behaviors, to achieve a particu-lar goal. It is essentially confidence that one can be successful in engaging in the planned course of action, that one can organize resources to achieve the goal and can overcome barriers when they occur.[80] Self-efficacy is fre-quently cited as a critical psychological mechanism that predicts successful weight management and increased physical activity[33] and is also noted in the pain management literature as important to successful pain manage-ment outcomes.[34] Improved self-efficacy during an intervention and main-tained postintervention has been shown to be associated with weight loss and physical activity,[81] and treatment approaches are increasingly includ-ing elements that directly target self-efficacy to improve behavioral adher-ence and weight loss outcomes.[82]

Cognitive models: Fear and avoidance

Pain catastrophizing, anxiety sensitivity, and pain related fear are com-monly identified as primary concepts in the fear avoidance model of pain. This model is a leading paradigm for understanding disability and chronic-ity associated with musculoskeletal pain and has wide support in cross-sectional, longitudinal, and experimental research.[83,84] Evidence suggests these concepts have further relevance to understanding adherence to phys-ical activity and weight loss.

The fear avoidance model of pain is a positive-feedback model that sug-gests two divergent sets of emotional, cognitive, and behavioral responses following acute pain. Depending on which responses are activated, an indi-vidual may either enter a cycle of confrontation coping or a cycle of exac-erbated and ongoing pain and disability. The first occurs when acute pain is perceived as nonthreatening and there is low fear and anxiety for the pain experienced, daily activities continue, and functional ability is main-tained. The second occurs when acute pain is interpreted catastrophically, which leads to pain-related fear and anxiety. Catastrophic misinterpreta-tions of pain can cause an excessive fear of pain and fear of activities that may cause pain (kinesiophobia). These fears eventually may generalize to a fear of physical movement, which leads to disuse, disability, and more pain. Anxiety sensitivity—a generalized fear of anxiety-related sensa-tions due to the belief that they may have harmful consequences—may contribute to pain either by magnifying fear or through its effect on pain catastrophizing.[85]

Individuals who demonstrate elevated anxiety sensitivity and catastrophizing about their pain may engage in a variety of avoidance coping behaviors. These may include eating during emotional stress and avoidance of physical activity, which will contribute to weight gain, increased pain, and poor health. Those with higher BMIs who demonstrate high levels of pain catastrophizing are at risk for higher levels of binge eating and lower self-efficacy for controlling eating behavior.[86] Pain catastrophizing and anxiety sensitivity have been shown to mediate the relationship between persistent pain and the likelihood to eat during emotional distress.[87] Individuals with pain who are prone to using food to cope with negative affect and provide pleasurable comfort may need additional strategies to aid them in managing negative emotions and self-soothing in order to be successful with long-term weight management. Unfortunately, observed changes in eating behavior may occur alongside decreased physical activity due to fear of pain and injury. Pain catastrophizing contributes to physical disability, potentially through its effect on self-efficacy for physical activity.[88] Individuals with high anxiety sensitivity are also more likely to be fearful during exercise,[89] fears that may lead them to avoid physical activity altogether. Individuals with pain and elevated BMI may be particularly more likely to perceive themselves as less able to engage in physical activity and more fearful of physical activity than nonobese peers.[90]

As there is a positive relationship between fear avoidance beliefs and disability in individuals with pain,[91] treatments that address these beliefs appear to have better outcomes than those that do not.[92] Addressing fear avoidance behaviors in individuals with pain and obesity may be especially important,[93] and both exposure-based and cognitive approaches may be efficacious.

Social and Environmental Domain

The environment in which one lives and the interpersonal interactions that occur within that environment have a significant impact on adherence to health behaviors. Models of behavior change often describe the importance of cues from and interactions with others as important factors influencing patient motivation and subsequent adherence to a particular health behavior. While these are often described as proximal interpersonal interactions that influence behavior, for example a HCP directly influencing a patient or a parent modeling a behavior for a child, we now know that more distal social and environmental factors also influence adherence to weight loss and physical activity.

Social networks

Obesity is a disorder that spreads through one's social network—if those around an individual are obese, then he or she is more likely to also be obese.[94] Social norms influence our health behaviors, dictating not only which health behavior goals we choose to pursue but also our adherence to these goals. For example, individuals with obesity who have more over-weight friends and who belong to a social network with more social accept-ability for unhealthy eating experience less weight loss during treatment.[95] In group treatment for weight loss, treatment adherence, including atten-dance at group sessions, use of meal replacements, and minutes of physi-cal activity, all appear to cluster within particular treatment groups.[96] This suggests that group norms develop over the course of treatment that influ-ence the likelihood of whether any one individual in the group adheres to the treatment plan.

Social networks have a powerful influence on individual behavior and thus are important to understand and improve adherence and treatment outcomes. Individuals are far less likely to be adherent to a plan to engage in weight loss or physical activity if individuals in their social network do not provide a context that supports these behaviors. Accordingly, obesity interventions are increasingly targeting social-relational constructs in intervention design, most commonly incorporating social support into treatment protocols,[97] which also is applicable to pain management. Other areas of health behavior change have demonstrated the utility of target-ing social networks to improve long-term treatment outcomes.[98] In these models individuals work to change their social network to include those who promote healthy behaviors, thus assisting them to create a social net-work supportive of healthful behavior change. The persuasive evidence that supports the importance of social networks to behavior, the potential for change in these networks to influence treatment outcomes, and the call from national leaders to understand and address social networks that pro-mote obesity[99] will likely increase the focus on social networks in behavior change in both obesity research and other areas of national health crises such as pain.

Environmental supports

Patient adherence to health behaviors occurs not only with in social net-works but also within the broader environmental context of their work and home neighborhoods. This environmental landscape is an important context for understanding adherence. The physical places where an individual spends his or her time are linked to health outcomes across multiple disease states.[100] For those with obesity, an individual's environment appears to influence not only weight status[101] but also the likelihood of engaging in behaviors that lead to long-term weight management.

The "obesogenic environment" is often characterized by variables that influence both physical activity and food consumption, although the impact of these factors appears to vary by neighborhood income such that individuals in low-socioeconomic neighborhoods are at especially increased risk.[102] Environments with reduced access to facilities that encourage physical activity and that fail to promote active modes of transportation (walking, biking) and recreation (parks, playgrounds) have lower rates of physical activity and higher rates of obesity.[103,104] Similarly, the availability of healthy foods and abundant supermarkets and fewer fast-food outlets has been shown associated with lower BMI.[103,105]

To directly address issues with the built and food environments typically requires large-scale policy change. This presents unique challenges to studying their effects. As a result, there are significant gaps in our understanding of effective environmental strategies to manage weight and increase physical activity. However, overall it appears interventions to alter the built environment can influence rates of physical activity. Similarly, interventions to address the food environment can change behaviors related to unhealthy food consumption, yet the overall impact on BMI remains less clear.[106]

INCREASING ADHERENCE TO WEIGHT LOSS FOR THE PATIENT WITH PAIN

Evidence-Based Recommendations for Weight Management

In 2013, the National Heart, Lung and Blood Institute of the National Institutes of Health appointed an expert panel to update the 1998 Clinical Guidelines on the Identification, Evaluation, and Treatment of Overweight and Obesity in Adults. This collaborative panel was formed with representatives from the American College of Cardiology, the American Heart Association Task Force on Practice Guidelines, and the Obesity Society and published their findings in the 2013 AHA/ACC/TOS Guideline for the Management of Overweight and Obesity in Adults.[6] The panel reviewed and evaluated data relevant to risk for obesity and overweight, benefits of weight loss, and treatment approaches to achieving weight loss. These areas were chosen based on their importance and relevance to clinical providers and the quality of the evidence. The panel's rigorous vetting of available evidence produced a document that outlines the current evidence-based standards of clinical practice with regard to weight management. Other relevant guidelines disseminated in 2014 include those published by the Department of Veterans Affairs' *Clinical Practice Guideline for Screening and Management of Overweight and Obesity*[107] and the National Institute for Health and Care Excellence (NICE) clinical guideline *Obesity: Identification, Assessment and Management.*[108] As the treatments outlined in these guidelines are those to which all clinicians should be encouraging patient adherence, these documents provide an important context for the approaches discussed in this chapter and are briefly summarized here.

The potential impact of obesity on the initiation and maintenance of persistent pain is underappreciated in clinical practice and underexamined by researchers.[109] This is curious given that for certain pain conditions obesity is a clear and significant risk factor. Accordingly, several pain management guidelines recommend weight management for control and prevention of pain disorders, particularly osteoarthritis.[110,111] Because of the significant body of research suggesting an association between obesity and lower limb osteoarthritis and evidence that weight maintenance or loss can reduce the incidence, progression, and impact of osteoarthritis, weight is clearly a clinical issue that should be addressed by HCPs with all patients who have osteoarthritis of the knee and hip. Increasingly, other pain conditions are shown to be highly correlated with obesity—for example, low back pain, which is the most prevalent type of pain. Since obesity is a significant public health issue with clear implications for morbidity, mortality, and patient quality of life and has been demonstrated to potentially negatively influence patient engagement in pain management,[41] all HCPs treating a patient for pain should address issues regarding weight whenever feasible and to the extent of their professional competence. While not every HCP will be able to offer comprehensive weight management, at a minimum all HCPs should be prepared to identify patient needs regarding weight management, refer patients to such care, collaborate with weight management providers, and support patients in the necessary changes required to improve health and weight.

Measuring Weight in Clinical Practice

BMI and waist circumference are recommended, practical approaches to weight assessment in clinical settings. BMI is calculated by dividing an individual's weight in kilograms by the square of their height in meters (kg/m^2). Overweight is classified as a BMI 25 to 29.9 kg/m^2; obesity is classified as a BMI $\geq$ 30 kg/m^2. These cut points are associated with elevated health risk and, in the case of obesity, all-cause mortality.[6]

Waist circumference is a useful measure of abdominal fat that is associated with increased health risk. Recommendations on specific cut points for waist circumference generally suggest that a waist circumference >102 cm among men and >88 cm among women is high and associated with greater risk.[6]

What Treatment, for Whom and When?

Evidence clearly suggests a dose-response relationship between increasing BMI and a number of health concerns, including cancer, cardiovascular disease, type 2 diabetes, osteoarthritis, pain, and all-cause mortality.[4] There is a relationship between increasing BMI and risk for persistent pain.[9] Lifestyle changes that produce even modest, sustained weight loss of 3% to 5% are associated with health benefits. Published guidelines recommend routine BMI screening of all patients, for those who are overweight or obese a discussion of risks associated with elevated BMI, and then at least annual assessment of waist circumference.

Clinical decisions regarding treatment initiation should be based on assessments of BMI, waist circumference, and obesity-related comorbidities. Other relevant information includes the patient's history of weight loss and current motivation for particular weight-relevant goals. Depending on their clinical history, current weight and health status, and motivation, current guidelines suggest patients should either be offered (a) lifestyle counseling using behavioral strategies or (b) bariatric surgery.

HCPs should consider providing all patients, even those of normal weight, information and behavioral counseling about healthy diet and physical activity behaviors in order to pursue/maintain a healthy weight. Such information may be a particularly important prevention strategy for individuals with persistent pain; as discussed, pain is a risk factor for weight gain. Information and behavioral counseling about diet and activity should also be offered to individuals with a BMI in the overweight range but who do not have any obesity-related comorbidities at the time of assessment and/or who do not have a high waist circumference.

Individuals who have a BMI in the overweight range and who also have obesity-related comorbidities or who demonstrate a high waist circumference should be recommended to participate in a long-term ($\geq$6 months), intensive ($\geq$14 sessions) comprehensive lifestyle program. These programs should be designed to help an individual lower daily caloric intake and increase physical activity using behavioral strategies led by a trained interventionist.

Individuals who have already lost weight but remain overweight or obese should be encouraged to participate in long-term (≥1 year) comprehensive weight loss maintenance program. These programs should include regular contact (at least monthly) with a trained interventionist to encourage ongoing high levels of physical activity, regular monitoring of body weight, and a reduced-calorie diet to maintain lower body weight.

Bariatric surgery may be an appropriate option for adults with a BMI ≥40 or a BMI ≥35 with obesity-related comorbid conditions who are motivated to lose weight but have not responded to behavioral treatment with sufficient weight loss to achieve a patient-specific targeted health outcome goal. Referral to an experienced bariatric surgeon for evaluation should be made for these patients.

Lifestyle Interventions for Weight Loss

Lifestyle interventions for weight loss as recommended by current practice guidelines include three key elements: (a) a reduced-calorie diet, (b) increased physical activity, and (c) behavior change to help facilitate adherence to diet and activity recommendations.

Reduced-calorie diet

The majority of lifestyle interventions prescribe a diet designed to induce a ≥500 kcal/day energy deficit, and there are several approaches used to achieve this goal. Perhaps the most straightforward is the prescription of 1200 to1500 kcal/day for women and 1500 to 1800 kcal/day for men. A more tailored approach calculates daily energy requirements based on sex, weight, and age using an equation such as the Harris Benedict Equation,[112] and this information forms the basis of an energy-deficit prescription. Finally, some approaches do not set an explicit target for a calorie deficit but rather advise individuals to avoid certain kinds of foods or to only eat certain foods or provide the food required for the prescribed diet. At this time comparative evidence is not available to prescribe which dietary approach will work best and for whom. A variety of dietary approaches have been shown to be effective at achieving weight loss, and no one approach appears more effective than the other.

Physical activity

Comprehensive interventions typically advise patients to increase aerobic physical activity to help increase energy expenditure.[6] Specific types of aerobic activity may vary depending on interest, ability, availability, and preference and may include both lifestyle changes (walking more, taking the stairs) or structured activities (home or gym-based fitness activities). Options offered should include both short intermittent bouts of activity (≥ 10 minutes) as well as longer continuous exercise. Current guidelines recommend ≥150 minutes per week of moderate-intensity physical activity to promote weight, averaging ≥30 minutes a day on most days of the week. Longer weekly durations of moderate-intensity physical activity (200–300 minutes per week) are recommended to maintain lost weight or minimize weight regain.[113] For the patient with chronic pain, achieving these goals may be more challenging. Initially it may be prudent to enlist the assistance of a physical therapist to design an exercise program that accommodates the individual patient's pain condition.

Behavioral strategies

A number of behavioral strategies are integrated into comprehensive lifestyle approaches to weight management, usually as a means to support diet and activity goals. Self-monitoring is often a key behavior to aid patients in tracking food intake, physical activity, and weight in order to meet prescribed goals, and frequency of tracking may vary from daily (for diet and activity) to weekly (for weight). Other techniques may include goal-setting, stimulus control, problem-solving, cognitive restructuring, relapse prevention, slowed rate of eating, and social support. These techniques are emphasized to varying degrees depending on the particular intervention, are often used in combination, and should be integrated into an individual approach for weight loss as appropriate for the patient.

Surgical interventions for weight loss

While referral to a bariatric surgeon is recommended by the most widely used guidelines for adults with a BMI ≥40 or a BMI ≥35 with obesity-related comorbid conditions, at this time there are no clear, guideline-based recommendations about the choice of specific bariatric surgical procedure. Outcomes and procedure selection may be impacted by patient factors, risk for complications, behavioral and psychosocial factors, and provider factors. Guidelines underscore the importance of patient commitment to long-term follow up and tracking of patient adherence to postsurgical lifestyle changes.[107,108]

The Patient–Provider Relationship: The Basis for Weight Loss Adherence and Motivation

Patients with persistent pain recognize the struggle to remain adherent to the complicated behavioral changes required for weight management and require help from their HCPs to maintain motivation.[114] Patient-centered care has been identified as critical to successful pain management,[115] and it is equally important for achieving patient adherence to weight management.[116] HCPs interactions with their patients provide an important context to encourage patient motivation for and adherence to the behaviors that support optimal health and weight management. HCPs are in a unique position to understand and assist patients in addressing the complex physiological, intrapersonal, and social factors that influence weight loss. As part of the patient's social and environmental domain, HCPs engage in behaviors that directly influence intrapersonal and behavioral factors that promote motivation and adherence. Some of these behaviors, such as facilitating working alliance via empathy and understanding, support adherence while others, such as being insensitive to the negative impact of weight stigma, serve as barriers to patient engagement and change.

Working Alliance

A positive working alliance between patient and HCP influences patient adherence and treatment outcome. Such an alliance is particularly important for individuals with pain and weight concerns as they are likely to describe clinical experiences that feel disrespectful and violate their trust in HCPs.[117,118] The working alliance between patient and HCP can be described as the degree to which both agree on the goals of treatment, both agree on the tasks each party will engage in to achieve the goals of treatment, and the bond that develops between the two characterized by mutual liking and trust.[119]

The importance of a working alliance on intrapersonal and behavioral factors has been well studied and is one of the most consistent and reliable predictors of patient outcomes across all forms of psychological treatment.[120] A positive working alliance has also been identified as one of the key aspects of patient-centered medical care.[121] Patient adherence and satisfaction with care are associated with a positive working alliance,[122] and working alliance predicts patients' adherence self-efficacy and perceptions of treatment utility.[123]

There are several communication skills HCPs can use to build an effective working alliance and increase trust, mutual goal-setting, and agreement on tasks.[124] Both verbal and nonverbal behaviors can contribute to trust and build rapport. HCPs should show empathy with the patient's circumstances, demonstrating that they understand the patient's view of their condition and the impact it has on their life. They should address the patient with compassion, honesty, and respect and treat them as a partner in the decision-making process, such that goals are identified and agreed upon mutually. Patients with pain and weight concerns may feel few HCPs understand or have concern for this comorbidity and impact it has on their health and quality of life. Patients should be given the opportunity to express their questions and concerns related to their pain and weight and provided with consistent and coordinated messages across a care team. The HCP should also discuss the extent to which the patient desires involvement from family and other significant sources of social support for their weight management.

Motivational interviewing

Motivational interviewing (MI) is a collaborative, patient-centered counseling approach that includes strategies likely to facilitate a working alliance.[125] MI is designed to promote motivation in individuals who are ambivalent about changing a behavior. MI is associated with improved pain adherence[126] and weight management adherence and outcomes.[127] Strategies associated with MI may influence intrapersonal and behavioral factors associated with adherence to weight loss and has been implemented by a variety of HCPs to promote weight loss in clinical settings.[127]

MI emphasizes two active components of HCPs relationships with patients: (a) a relational component focused on empathy, interpersonal process, and understanding of the patient's perspective and (b) a technical component that involves promoting discrepancy and reinforcement of change talk.[128] A goal of MI is to help patients find their own solutions to problems and foster internal motivation to change. MI-consistent behaviors could include reinforcement and praise ("That's great that you are trying to stop drinking soda"), collaboration ("What can I do to help you meet your daily walking goal?"), and statements that help evoke change talk from the patient ("What might be some good things that come from being more physically active?"). From an MI perspective, advice is not given without first making sure the patient wants to hear suggestions, and HCPs should never judge, criticize, or directly confront patients about their behaviors in a way that violates patient respect and autonomy.

Provider Attitude toward Obesity and Weight Loss: Understanding and Addressing Bias to Facilitate Adherence

HCPs attitudes toward weight loss and obesity have a significant effect on patient adherence and may alter a patient's working alliance with an individual HCP and trust of HCPs generally. Changing weight stigma in healthcare addresses a potentially important barrier to weight loss and adherence in a patient's social and environmental domain. Weight stigma violates patient respect and autonomy and may reduce the quality of care provided and cause avoidance of care, mistrust, and poor adherence among individuals with obesity.[129] Weight bias has been documented across a wide range of health professionals, including physicians, psychologists, nurses, and fitness professionals. Physician attitudes about people with obesity tend to be negative, and these attitudes directly and negatively influence clinical encounters with patients who are obese.[129] There is also a high likelihood for individuals with persistent pain to experience stigma in healthcare settings.[117] This leaves patients with both pain and weight concerns at double the risk for negative experiences. The Rudd Center for Food Policy & Obesity (www.uconnruddcenter.org) provides excellent tools to aid clinicians in identifying and addressing weight stigma in clinical practice, and several recommendations are summarized here.

Self-assessment

All HCPs should engage in self-assessment about their attitudes regarding patients who are obese and patients who have pain, and especially patients with co-occurring pain and obesity, to uncover and address potential bias. There are a number of well-validated instruments that can be used either for self-assessment or group training activities to examine and discuss weight bias in clinical practice, including an Implicit Associations Test,[130] the Fat Phobia Scale,[131] the Antifat Attitudes Scale, the Attitudes About Obese Persons Scale,[132] and the Beliefs About Obese Persons Scale.[133]

Education

Accurate information can reduce obesity prejudice. HCPs who have accurate information on the complex factors that contribute to obesity have more positive attitudes toward patients with obesity compared to those who understand obesity as a disorder of simply consuming too many calories combined with too little caloric burn.[129] Such education is important for all individuals providing direct clinical services but should also occur at the appropriate level to help clerical and administrative staff understand the unique challenges facing individuals with higher BMIs and persistent pain. Clinics should have a clearly defined policy regarding comments and/ or humor that stereotypes anyone based on a physical attribute or disability and a plan for remediation when violations occur.

Clinic environment

Practices should examine their office environments to determine how accommodating they are to individuals who have higher BMIs. Many of the accessibility concerns for individuals who are overweight are likely shared by individuals with persistent pain. For example, are chairs of the appropriate size and construction for an individual to sit comfortably? Will the diagnostic and assessment tools available (e.g., scales, blood pressure cuffs, exam tables) accommodate patients with heavier weights? Are reading materials offered in the clinic setting likely to make the person with pain and weight concerns more body-conscious? Are hand-rails, ramps, and other assistive devices installed in their proper places? Also, assessments of the office and clinic environments should be included as part of patient feedback. The American Medical Association has a helpful checklist for HCPs to aid them in assessing their clinic space for accessibility and comfort for patients with obesity.[134]

Clinical interactions

In clinical interactions, the focus on body weight should be reduced and the focus on encouraging behaviors that improve health and well-being overall emphasized. Evidence suggests that a weight-inclusive approach— one that emphasizes health as multifaceted and the ability of one to be "Healthy at Every Size"—can improve outcomes in several health-related domains and is likely to increase patient adherence to health-promoting behavioral strategies (e.g., increased physical activity).[135] Providers should choose language carefully and avoid language that is stigmatizing or blaming. Terms like "unhealthy weight" and "BMI" are preferred over more stigmatizing terms such as "fat" and "morbidly obese."[136]

The Five A's of Behavior Change: A Framework to Facilitate Weight Loss Adherence

Newly revised obesity treatment guidelines include a treatment approach based on the Five A's (5As) framework for facilitating change—Assess, Advise, Agree, Assist, and Arrange.[6] HCP advice about weight loss has a significant impact on patient attempts to change weight-related behaviors. For these reasons, we encourage all pain providers to engage patients in brief counseling about weight loss and, when appropriate, referral to and coordination with other providers. The 5As is a brief counseling model that, when used by HCPs, can increase patient motivation to lose weight, improve their diet, and exercise.[137] Use of the 5As to address obesity in clinical settings appears to strengthen patient–HCP communication,[138] and appropriate use of all strategies outlined by the framework can positively improve patient motivation for and adherence to weight loss.[139]

Ask: Assessment Is Key to Successful Weight Management in the Patient with Pain

Many individuals who set out to manage their weight through lifestyle change eventually reduce or discontinue the lifestyle changes and ultimately regain any weight lost. Dropout rates from weight loss interventions have been reported as high as 80%, and unrealistic expectations about and goals for weight loss appear related to dropout.[140] Individuals with pain are particularly likely to struggle with weight loss treatment.[30] Accurate assessment aids the HCP in identifying relevant physiological, behavioral, and environmental factors that may undermine adherence, and choosing target behaviors and goals based on this assessment and patient's readiness to change can facilitate adherence. Once identified, barriers can provide important information to help HCPs achieve other clinical tasks critical to promoting adherence and weight loss success, including advising patients on risks associated with higher BMIs, setting appropriate goals for treatment, and assisting patients in addressing problems when they occur.

Motivation and the Transtheoretical Model

Readiness to change describes a patient's motivation to engage in particular behaviors during a specific timeframe. Providers can help their patients achieve weight loss by applying motivational techniques that encourage adherence by targeting a treatment approach to the patient's readiness to change. The Transtheoretical Model (TTM) is based on the concept of readiness to change and stages of change and can complement MI-based approaches. It provides a theoretical framework to aid the provider in determining readiness to change and matching a tailored intervention according to the patient's motivation for weight management.[141] The TTM describes the relationships between stages of change—precontemplation, contemplation, preparation, action, and maintenance—and the process of change across these stages.[142] Individuals may move through the stages of change in any manner, and these stages are related to specific needs with regard to decision-making about behavior change and self-efficacy.

The stages of change are defined broadly according to the individual's readiness to engage in change during a specific period of time. In the precontemplation stage, individuals are not considering weight loss within the next six months. Some in this stage may be entirely uninterested in weight management while others may wish to delay addressing weight. At this stage, provider approaches that highlight and personalize the potential health risks of weight and benefits of healthy lifestyle change may be appropriate. However, typically the patient is not ready to receive information on specific change strategies. The contemplation stage is characterized by individuals considering changes to address weight during the upcoming six months. Individuals in this stage are often receptive to information regarding weight and health and strategies to address weight concerns. The preparation stage is characterized by an increasing commitment towards weight loss and preparing to address their weight within the next month or so. During this stage, individuals can benefit from HCPs who help them solidify their commitment and plans for change. Information regarding specific strategies and referrals to resources may be useful. In the action stage individuals are actively working to address their weight and have begun to do so within the past six months. Individuals at this stage may need support, reinforcement, and help with problem-solving their weight loss behaviors and assistance addressing obstacles and preventing relapse. During the maintenance stage, an individual has worked to address weight for at least the past six months. Typically, the behavioral changes associated with weight loss are now more habitual. Relapse is still a risk that needs to be addressed, but the risk becomes less during this stage than previous stages.

Assessing readiness to change

To assess readiness to change, HCPs should inquire about a patents awareness of the problem, willingness to change, and the actions they believe necessary to make the specific change. Weight loss is a complex behavior that involves changing of multiple behaviors simultaneously. Patients may be more ready to change one behavior than another. Standardized assessment approaches for readiness to change weight have good reliability and validity, and multi-item assessments may be at times advantageous[143]; however, in the clinical setting single-question assessments of target behaviors may be more practical and equally helpful to guide treatment.[144] Using this approach, a HCP asks how ready a patient is to engage in a specific target behavior such as increasing planned exercise, increasing daily activity, increasing fruit or vegetable consumption, and decreasing portion size. This approach can help to successfully identify target behaviors for which the patient has more readiness and motivation to engage, and thus these are more promising targets for change. This allows the HCP to target efforts toward behaviors to which a patient is most likely to adhere and thus might have the most significant impact on weight management.

Assessing psychosocial characteristics and comorbidities

An important advantage of the 5As model is that it reminds the HCP to assess not only patient's readiness to make a behavior change but also other areas such as comorbidities that may interfere with weight loss. Persistent pain is a comorbidity associated with attenuated weight loss outcomes.[30] Assessment in patients with pain should occur across the domains likely to influence adherence and motivation so the HCP may identify potential physiological, intrapersonal/behavioral, and social/environmental factors that influence adherence. In particular, a thorough pain assessment is the foundation for a weight management plan in the person with pain. Physical limitations associated with the patient's pain presentation or other medical conditions should be addressed and integrated into any plans for weight management. There are a number of conditions that present a high risk for weight loss failure that frequently co-occur with pain disorders, including depression, binge eating, and sleep disorders; these should be assessed and comanaged during treatment to optimize goal selection and maximize adherence. Of these, current research suggests depression appears particularly relevant to both pain, obesity, and the co-occurrence of the two.

Depression

There is a significant body of literature suggesting separately that both obesity[145] and pain[146] are associated with symptoms of depression, and pain has been shown to be worse among obese individuals with depression.[147] Depression is associated with higher caloric intake,[148] and depressive symptoms are correlated with an increased likelihood of eating during negative mood (emotional or stress-induced eating) and lower engagement in and self-efficacy for physical activity.[148,149] In individuals with persistent pain and obesity, depression increases the likelihood that they will not adhere to healthy behaviors (exercise, proper nutrition) that could contribute to positive outcomes for both pain and weight management.[32] Accordingly, depression should be assessed in the patient with pain and weight concerns, and when depression is identified it should be addressed alongside weight and pain concerns.

Advise: Tailored Information to Promote Weight Loss Success

HCP advice should focus on a personalized discussion of risks associated with unhealthful behaviors/increased weight and the benefits of behavior change to mitigate these risks and improve health. This advice should be evidence-based yet tailored to the patient. The goal of this advice is to aid the patient in understanding his or her unique health concerns related to weight and health behaviors. For patients who do not demonstrate current readiness to change, accurate and tailored advice may also help facilitate movement to a stage where they are willing to contemplate or engage in change.

HCPs should discuss the risks of increased weight using language that is tailored to the patient's current weight and health status, pain, and risk for specific conditions. Advice should be guided by one's expertise and competencies. Persistent pain is a very clear risk factor associated with increased weight. Thus beginning discussions with an overview of the relationship between pain and weight likely provides a natural starting point for HCP advice. Be specific with patients regarding how weight may impact their pain and how weight loss may benefit their pain. Patients should be counseled that even modest weight loss is associated with significant health benefits. For individuals with persistent pain conditions, weight loss is associated with reduced disability. Maximal benefit for pain symptoms is achieved when weight loss is greater than 5% of baseline body weight.[22,26]

To achieve weight loss, patients should be encouraged to reduce their caloric intake approximately 500 to 1,000 calories each day.[6] Clinicians should be aware that patients with pain may be particularly inactive, thus planned energy deficits may need to be greater to help compensate,[23] but this may be challenging depending on the extent of the patient's disabilities. Generally, a calorie deficit can be achieved in any manner that is agreeable to the patient and matches his or her current readiness to change; however, patients should be advised that the optimal approach is one that includes dietary changes and increased physical activity. Furthermore, caloric intake should be appropriately distributed among nutrients to minimize loss of bone density and lean muscle mass that may particularly impact the patient with pain[23,150]; if possible, a consult with a nutritionist will likely be beneficial. Both short- and long-term studies suggest that dietary changes and exercise used in combination help patients with pain and obesity achieve improved weight loss, improved physical function, and increased mobility compared to approaches that focus on exercise, diet, or rehabilitation alone.[151] One study examining the effects of diet and exercise compared to either approach alone found the combined treatment demonstrated less inflammation, less pain, better function, faster walking speed, and better health-related quality of life.[26] Thus dietary change plus exercise appears to produce more consistent, long-term improvements in physical function, biological and mechanical markers, and psychosocial outcomes in individuals with pain along with weight loss.

Agree: Setting and Adhering to Goals for Weight Management

Setting goals and helping patients meet these goals is important to achieve behavioral change and adherence,[152] yet providers often spend too little time working toward goal agreement with their patients.[153] Patients interested in weight loss often want to set a specific level of weight loss as a goal; however, there is considerable debate about whether these goals should be realistic (e.g., 5% weight loss) or aspirational (e.g., > 15% weight loss). Some evidence suggests a realistic weight loss goal is preferable; other evidence suggests that setting realistic weight loss goals does not facilitate weight loss[154] and that less realistic goals may be associated with better weight loss.[42] Given these discrepancies, HCPs should focus on the specific behaviors associated with weight management and health rather than a specific unit of weight loss to achieve.

Weight loss or maintenance may be the desired outcome, but goals should be focused around patient behavioral targets. Focusing on the behaviors that contribute to weight loss, rather than the weight loss itself, has been shown to promote weight loss and feelings of behavioral mastery.[155] Focusing on healthy behavioral changes like diet and physical activity also allows the HCP to highlight how such changes may positively impact not only weight status but also pain status. Indeed, ideally such conversations should take place as part of the discussion regarding the patient's overall treatment plan. The patient should not feel as if there are disparate, competing goals—some to address pain and others to address weight. Rather, patients should perceive that the goals set will be ones that will improve their health overall and are part of the treatment program to address pain.

Goal-setting should be a collaborative process driven by the patient's specific needs. A common approach is setting goals that are Specific, Measurable, Attainable, Relevant, and Time-Based (SMART). Goals should identify specific behaviors to change during a specific timeframe and should be reasonable given the patient's pain status, comorbidities, and social/ environmental constraints. Goals should be relevant to achieving weight loss in the context of pain management. Patients and providers should be able to measure goal progress and, thus, assess progress to achieving the goal. For example, a SMART goal is, "I will walk for 15 minutes four times each week" rather than "I want to exercise more."

HCPs should work with patients on identifying tools and techniques necessary to achieve their goals. If patients do not have the skills or resources needed to achieve the goal, the goal is not a helpful one. HCPs should have a plan to provide referral to specific providers or resources for patients. Self-monitoring is often a helpful tool for patients attempting weight loss to track their progress and provide feedback. Patients should be encouraged to use the self-monitoring approach that works best for them. For some, this may be tracking on pen and paper or using a small pocket notebook. For many others, it may include use of commercial mobile or web-based applications to aid in monitoring dietary intake, physical activity, and weight. These applications often include goal-setting, and their use can be helpful for achieving weight loss.[156] Tools are also available to help providers assess and recommend useful mobile applications.[157] It may be helpful for patients to monitor these behavioral changes alongside relevant pain targets, like intensity and interference. Collected data can be reviewed with the patient to facilitate discussion about progress, reassess goals, and problem-solve barriers.

Assist: Common Barriers and Approaches to Problem-Solving

An important role for the pain provider is to assist both patients and other providers in understanding how to appropriately tailor weight management strategies to meet the needs of patients with pain. Patients with pain report feeling discouraged that informational materials offered to aid them in weight loss are not adequately tailored to their pain complaints and personal history.[114] HCPs should work with patient to identify barriers and aid them in problem-solving to address these barriers with specific strategies. Barriers may occur in a number of domains and include physiological, intrapersonal/behavioral, or social/environmental concerns. HCPs can offer an important source of encouragement and problem-solving that can have a positive impact of self-efficacy for weight loss. Some patients may require more intensive behavioral counseling and support, and current guidelines recommend intensive treatment to achieve and maintain weight loss.[6] Thus HCPs should consider referral for these patients to a behavioral psychologist or other specialist provider or program for weight management support if other providers have not already made such referrals.

Self-efficacy and pain catastrophizing

Patients who demonstrate poorer pain coping may be particularly at risk for attenuated weight management outcomes. Individuals with higher levels of pain catastrophizing appear likely to have higher BMIs along with greater pain severity and lower self-efficacy.[158] Individuals with obesity who report high pain catastrophizing are also more likely to demonstrate binge eating and lower self-efficacy for controlling eating behavior.[86] Pain catastrophizing may influence patient outcome via domain-specific self-efficacy, such that domain-specific self-efficacy may mediate the impact of catastrophizing on the associated outcome.[88] Cognitive approaches that address catastrophizing and increase positive emotions, optimism, and hope are effective; even brief interventions that help patients understand the biopsychosocial model of pain, the impact of thoughts on pain response, and basic tools for coping can be effective.[159]

Self-efficacy is important for understanding weight management in individuals with persistent pain as it appears that specific health-related thoughts are related to specific outcomes. Patients who have low self-efficacy may struggle to adhere to dietary recommendations and physical activity goals. Domain-specific self-efficacy can predict outcome in individuals with pain and weight concerns[88] and points to the need for HCPs to assess self-efficacy for specific areas to address in treatment. While self-efficacy for arthritis, for example, can predict physical functioning and performance on physical assessments, self-efficacy for weight management can predict overeating.[160] Self-efficacy for pain and weight management behaviors should be monitored, and there are a number of brief measures that could be used in clinical practice.[161] HCPs can help improve self-efficacy by making sure patients understand specifically how they are to perform target behaviors and how to make adjustments to address their pain by providing training directly, offering an appropriate model, or referring to others to help provide the necessary skill training.

Environmental and social support

Patients with pain and weight concerns report they do not feel comfortable in traditional workout environments, in part due to concerns about body image and pain limitations. Other research supports the likelihood of patients with higher levels of pain to have disrupted body image.[162] Finding an environment where the patient with pain feels comfortable to be physically active is a barrier that HCPs can address by discussing with patients the specific environments that appeal to them and ways to use available resources to meet the patient's activity needs. Similarly, lack of social support for the many specific changes required to manage weight may also be an obstacle. Social support can aid behavioral weight loss, help with adherence after weight loss postbariatric surgery,[163] and attenuate pain and stress.[164] The challenge for the patient with pain and weight control issues is finding appropriate social support. Online "virtual" resources and mobile applications offer opportunities for support, as do community resources that connect patients with similar concerns.

Arrange: Making a Plan for Follow-Up

Patients with pain and weight concerns want their HCPs to help them access the resources needed to meet their goals and actively address their pain and weight concerns.[114] While pain providers can serve an important role in increasing adherence to weight loss, they may not have the time or training to deliver the intense level of intervention required to achieve significant and sustained weight loss. Intensive behavioral treatment is recommended as such treatment, partnered with primary or specialist HCP oversight through regular visits, is more likely to produce weight loss ≥ 5% of initial weight than physician counseling without additional support.[165]

Pain specialists should be prepared to offer appropriate referrals for weight management and to follow up with patients about this care and support weight loss efforts. They should collaborate with care providers and educate them on the potential limitations imposed by the patient's pain condition and take care to refer patients to colleagues known to understand the relationship between pain and weight. In particular, patients who are struggling with weight loss should be referred for more intensive counseling. HCPs should have a list of affordable community resources to help patients reach their goals and use the most recent obesity treatment guidelines to determine whether services provided are evidence-based. Community health centers, YMCAs, and community recreation facilities may all provide important, and often low-cost, resources. Once a referral has been made, providers should make a plan to follow up with the patient at a specific, mutually agreed-upon interval and subsequent intervals as appropriate.

INCREASING ADHERENCE TO PHYSICAL ACTIVITY FOR THE PATIENT WITH PAIN

Physical Activity as a First-Line Treatment for Pain

Across the world, clinical practice guidelines advocate physical activity as a first-line, nonpharmacologic treatment approach to the conservative management of many chronic pain conditions ranging from fibromyalgia to low back pain as well osteoarthritis of the knee, hip, and hands.[166,167] Compared to pharmacological treatment or surgery, physical activity interventions offer a less costly approach with little risk for serious adverse events.[168]

The main goals of evidence-based physical activity treatments are to reduce pain, improve physical function, and help patients resume normal participation in activities of daily living.[168,169] Physical activity treatments offer the advantage of directly addressing physiological impairments associated with many pain conditions by improving muscular strength, cardiorespiratory fitness, proprioception, balance, and mobility and reducing the risk for falls. Furthermore, physical activity is a nonpharmacological approach to addressing many physical and psychological symptoms of pain, including anxiety, depression, fatigue, poor sleep, and joint immobility.[167] However, maintaining adherence to an exercise program and a physically active lifestyle are essential to sustaining these clinical benefits over time.[168,170]

Defining the Elements of Evidence-Based Physical Activity Interventions

For both patients and providers, interpreting guideline recommendations can be confusing because the terms *physical activity* and *exercise* are used interchangeably, often without explanation. Current public health exercise guidelines such as those disseminated by the American College of Sports Medicine define *physical activity* as "Any bodily movement produced by skeletal muscles that results in energy expenditure above resting levels which, encompasses exercise, sports, and physical activities done as part of daily living, occupation, leisure, and active transportation."[113] Comparatively, *exercise* is defined as, "Physical activity that is planned, structured, and repetitive and that has a final or intermediate objective the improvement or maintenance of physical activity."[113] *Exercise* is the term used more commonly in guidelines largely because the evidence underlying these recommendations are based on clinical trials that used exercise protocols rather than unstructured lifestyle activities.

When developing an exercise/physical activity program, patients and HCPs should collaborate to agree on some fundamental components of the program, including the *type* of exercise/activity, *frequency* of activity per week, *intensity* of the activity, and *time* engaged in activity per day or episode of activity. Collectively, these components make up the "dose" of an exercise prescription, which can be tailored to the individual patient. Exercise and physical activity may be performed on land or water and may involve one or more *types* of exercise, including muscle strengthening/resistance training, cardiovascular/aerobic conditioning, stretching/range of motion exercises, and neuromuscular exercises like Tai Chi, yoga, and exercises to develop motor skills associated with balance, coordination, and gait.

Patients have a choice regarding where they participate in exercise based on a range of modes of exercise delivery that can include individually supervised sessions with a physiotherapist (PT) or exercise professional, supervised group-based sessions, or programs performed by the patient individually at home or at a community exercise facility, with or without the supervision of a PT or exercise professional. In clinical practice, most exercise programs for pain consist of a combination of these modalities, beginning with a supervised mode of delivery and transitioning to a home- or community-based program.[171] Although pain guidelines typically specify the type of exercise and delivery mode for different types of pain, recommendations are less precise regarding the exercise prescription elements of intensity, frequency, and total weekly activity.

Interpreting Exercise Guidelines for Patients with Chronic Pain

Clinical practice guidelines about the use of exercise for pain are somewhat ambiguous, as evidence from research studies has not yet revealed the optimal modality, intensity, duration, and/or frequency.[167,171] For HCPs, this can result in uncertainty regarding how to apply general guideline recommendations for physical activity/exercise to their patients with chronic pain who vary greatly in their abilities to perform exercise and are less likely to attain guideline goals.[172,173] General physical activity guidelines encourage adults to participate in a regular exercise program *beyond* their daily activities with the goals of (a) attaining at least 30 minutes/day of moderate to vigorous intensity aerobic activity for a total of 150 minutes/ week and (b) engaging in resistance training two to three times per week.

These targets are unrealistic for many pain patients, yet it is frequently overlooked that the general guidelines[113] acknowledge the need to modify exercise program goals to account for impairments based on physical function, health status, exercise response, and/or stated goals. Moreover, the guidelines emphasize that people with pain requiring modifications to their goals can still derive health benefits from engaging in levels of exercise less than recommended by engaging in shorter bouts (e.g., 10 minutes) of activity and avoid the deleterious effects accrued from a sedentary lifestyle. Indeed, evidence shows that patients with chronic pain may be more successful when they chose a lower intensity of exercise than the standard guidance. Specifically, exercise programs that start at a lower level of intensity and progress steadily tend not to exacerbate pain and stiffness and appear to result in greater exercise adherence, less program attrition, and greater gains in quality of life.[167]

The Evidence for Exercise Prescription for People with Chronic Pain

Systematic and meta-analytic reviews provide valuable insights about the relative benefit of specific exercise types and delivery modalities. First, there is considerable evidence to show the effects of land- and aquatic-based exercise on pain management for people with low back pain, fibromyalgia, rheumatoid arthritis, and various forms of osteoarthritis are comparable to those derived from simple analgesics and nonsteroidal anti-inflammatory drugs but without the potential iatrogenic harms of these medications.[174–178] Second, exercise therapy is not only beneficial for people with mild to moderate pain conditions but should include those with severe pain, such as those waiting total joint replacement surgery.[167,179] In some conditions, such as low back pain, exercise or exercise with education are effective in preventing episodes of pain.[180] Third, the benefits of cardiorespiratory and resistance exercises (land and aquatic-based) are comparable for reducing pain and improving function across pain conditions but optimized when both exercises are combined in a program with flexibility training.[175]

Despite consistent findings of short-term (less than six months) improvements associated with exercise interventions for pain, among the limited number of studies reporting long-term outcomes, results indicate that benefits decline over time related to nonadherence.[181,182] Conversely, evidence suggests that although individual exercise treatments, supervised group classes, and home-based exercise are all effective in reducing pain symptoms, the quality of HCP supervision may improve outcomes across these modalities to support adherence. In one meta-analysis, a comparison of studies where participants received fewer than 12 supervised sessions yielded small treatment effects for pain and function whereas studies with 12 or more supervised sessions demonstrated moderate treatment effects.[183] Given the complex and varied presentations of patients with chronic pain, a qualified professional can optimize exercise treatment outcomes by customizing an exercise program to meet the needs, goals, and interests of the patient.[168] Furthermore, supervision in the early stages of a class- or home-based program can reduce adverse events by helping participants adopt safe and correct exercise techniques and by appropriately matching the exercise dose to the participants' personal goals and abilities. However, use of general, untailored exercise programs that allow little room to address patient's personal limitations and pain symptoms have been found ineffective.[184]

Recommendations to Enhance Physical Activity with the Socioecological Model

Despite the existence of clinical practice guidelines advocating exercise and physical activity interventions as first-line, nonpharmacological treatment approaches for chronic pain, these recommendations have not been reliably and meaningfully implemented into regular practice by medical practitioners and allied health professionals.[185,186] Box 5.1 summarizes key recommendations to support exercise adherence for the pain patient at the patient, provider, and environmental level by proactively addressing multilevel barriers and factors affecting physical activity behavior over time.

Enabling HCPs to support exercise adherence is a critical step to making exercise treatment a more highly utilized pain management strategy in clinical practice settings. Historically, low uptake of clinical practice recommendations can be attributed to providers' knowledge, beliefs, attitudes, and behaviors toward physical activity/exercise. Prior cross-sectional studies indicate when HCPs lacked training in exercise prescription or current knowledge about specific treatment guidelines, research, or the availability

Box 5.1

RECOMMENDATIONS TO SUPPORT ADHERENCE IN PATIENTS WITH CHRONIC PAIN

- Providers should reinforce the message that exercise/physical activity is safe and an essential part of pain treatment and self-management for all types of chronic pain.
- Providers should emphasize that some activity, no matter how minimal in intensity and duration, is better than becoming inactive during acute pain flare-ups.
- Exercise prescription is an ongoing, shared decision-making process between patients and providers (primary care, pain, physiotherapist, exercise professional).
- Exercise programs should be individualized to account for a patient's age, mobility, comorbidities, knowledge, preferences, and access to exercise resources.
- Supervised programs should incorporate measurement-based care principles to assess specific impairments, health status, barriers to exercise, and psychosocial status at program entry, with regular follow-up to monitor treatment response and to make program adjustments to maintain motivation and program adherence.
- Providers should utilize strategies such as Motivational Interviewing, the 5As, and cognitive behavioral treatment to help activate patient motivational resources (social support, enjoyment), pain coping skills, and problem-solving barriers to participation and address psychosocial issues such as depression and anxiety.
- Exercise programming is optimized when augmented with education and advice about how to self-manage a particular pain condition through lifestyle behaviors (weight loss, physical activity) and coping strategies during acute episodes of pain.
- Effective exercise programs should involve both strengthening and aerobic exercises.
- High-intensity exercises should generally be discouraged for pain management.
- Some obese patients and those with higher pain severity may need to start with aquatic or nonweight-bearing exercises and gradually progress in intensity to avoid pain exacerbation.
- Exercise outcomes are enhanced when supervised by a trained physiotherapist or exercise professional, particularly when patients attend ≥ 12 sessions.
- Group and home-based exercise programs are equally effective and should follow an individualized program.
- Providers who are part of the same practice or health system and can coordinate care using a collaborative, patient-centered medical home model are better prepared to implement changes to support exercise adherence and link patients to effective community-based exercise professionals and programs.

of resources for patients, discussion about exercise treatments do not occur. Similarly, negative HCP attitudes and beliefs toward exercise undermine the likelihood that patients will have the opportunity to consider exercise as a pain management strategy. For example, in one US survey of 10,892 adults with osteoarthritis, respondents who said that their HCP recommended exercise to manage their disease were significantly more likely to exercise than those who had not received such a recommendation.[187]

A recent review of 16 international pain treatment guidelines for osteoarthritis attempted to harmonize and simplify treatment guidelines to enhance HCP use by using visual algorithms to highlight common clinical cases.[188] These algorithms call for HCPs to start treatment with conservative, nonpharmacologic procedures over more high-risk or invasive procedures. Clinical assessment starts with an examination of signs and symptoms of pain as well as review of any relevant medical or psychological comorbidities. The first step in treatment upon diagnosis is to encourage a patient to try one or more nonpharmacological behavioral treatment strategies, including (a) a weight program available in the community; (b) a community-based physical activity program, community exercise program, or home exercise program; and (c) a pain self-management and education program; and (d) psychological treatment such as cognitive behavioral therapy to assist with pain coping or comorbid psychological symptoms. If the HCP's examination finds the patient is weak, stiff, or has functional deficits, then it is appropriate to make a referral to a PT or occupational therapist for additional diagnostic assessment and to develop a personally tailored exercise program.

For these algorithms to be viable in practice, this model requires HCPs to be part of a network of providers or an integrated healthcare system that can facilitate coordination of care between medical providers and allied health professionals including the PT, mental health therapist, and preferably exercise professional.[189] National health care initiatives have incentivized HCPs to adopt healthcare delivery models such as the patient-centered medical homes and accountable care organizations to improve outcomes in patients with chronic conditions and minimize adverse events from pain medications.

With greater acceptance of guideline recommendations, allied health providers should be prepared to adopt a flexible and proactive approach to address potential patient issues pertaining to weight management and physical activity among patients referred who have pain.[171] People with chronic pain represent a complex population with varying limitations, clinical issues, and personal needs and goals. Thus HCPs, like physiotherapists and exercise professionals, should aim to initially identify patient's individual barriers and facilitating factors to exercise using screening tools[171,190,191] to augment their normal intake procedures. This information can be used to help the HCP propose exercise recommendations that are more appropriately tailored to a patient's physical capabilities and to propose strategies to help the patient overcome potential barriers and challenges. Successful exercise programs must avoid exacerbating pain, progress gradually until a plateau of fitness that can be maintained, and be feasible for a patient with respect to access to transportation, facilities, and available exercise equipment.[171]

As with weight loss change, the HCP should aim to use a variety of behavioral change strategies (such a problem-solving, goal setting) including use of the 5As and MI techniques to elicit and activate sources of social support, provide educational information, strengthen self-efficacy, and address negative thoughts, beliefs, attitudes, or cognitions about exercise or health concerns affecting exercise (such as depression, catastrophizing, insomnia, binge eating). To support adherence, providers should help patients find an exercise program that is enjoyable, accessible, and congruent with their goals and values. Given the many erroneous beliefs about exercise and pain, HCPs should educate patients[192,193] about the relationship between sedentary behavior and physical function, correct misconceptions about exercise (exercise does not have to be intense, can occur in short bouts versus long duration), share information about the benefits of an exercise program and what outcomes are realistic and assist patients in learning to monitor exercise intensity and recognize transient increases in pain or discomfort associated with exercise versus a serious exacerbation of pain.

CONCLUSIONS

Maintaining a healthy weight and engaging in regular physical activity are two health behaviors that will play an increasing role in the nonpharmacological treatment of chronic pain. Helping patients with chronic pain adhere to these lifestyle programs over time to sustain the benefits of weight loss and/or physical activity is challenging. We propose that a socioecological model of adherence to healthy lifestyle behaviors in individuals with pain can assist providers in understanding the physiological, intrapersonal/behavioral, and social/environmental factors that influence adherence. HCPs who tailor patient treatment programs at multiple levels can optimize adherence to weight loss and physical activity interventions by proactively identifying barriers and developing recommendations or strategies to support patients in overcoming these challenges.

REFERENCES

1. Ng M, Fleming T, Robinson M, et al. Global, regional, and national prevalence of overweight and obesity in children and adults during 1980–2013: a systematic analysis for the Global Burden of Disease Study 2013. *Lancet.* 2014;384(9945):766–781.

2. Flegal KM, Carroll MD, Kit BK, Ogden CL. Prevalence of obesity and trends in the distribution of body mass index among US adults, 1999–2010. *JAMA.* 2012;307(5):491–497.

3. Flegal KM, Kit BK, Orpana H, Graubard BI. Association of all-cause mortality with overweight and obesity using standard body mass index categories: a systematic review and meta-analysis. *JAMA.* 2013;309(1):71–82.

4. Guh DP, Zhang W, Bansback N, Amarsi Z, Birmingham CL, Anis AH. The incidence of co-morbidities related to obesity and overweight: a systematic review and meta-analysis. *BMC Public Health.* 2009;9:88.

5. Finkelstein EA, Trogdon JG, Cohen JW, Dietz W. Annual medical spending attributable to obesity: payer-and service-specific estimates. *Health Aff.* 2009;28(5):w822–w831.

6. Jensen MD, Ryan DH, Apovian CM, et al. 2013 AHA/ACC/TOS guideline for the management of overweight and obesity in adults: a report of the American College of Cardiology/American Heart Association Task Force on Practice Guidelines and the Obesity Society. *Circulation.* 2014;129(25 Suppl. 2):S102–S138.

7. Veerman JL, Barendregt JJ, van Beeck EF, Seidell JC, Mackenbach JP. Stemming the obesity epidemic: a tantalizing prospect. *Obesity.* 2007;15(9):2365–2370.

8. Janke EA, Collins A, Kozak AT. Overview of the relationship between pain and obesity: What do we know? Where do we go next? *J Rehabil Res Dev.* 2007;44(2):245–262.

9. Stone AA, Broderick JE. Obesity and pain are associated in the United States. *Obesity.* 2012;20(7):1491–1495.

10. Wright LJ, Schur E, Noonan C, Ahumada S, Buchwald D, Afari N. Chronic pain, overweight, and obesity: findings from a community-based twin registry. *J Pain.* 2010;11(7):628–635.

11. Frilander H, Solovieva S, Mutanen P, Pihlajamaki H, Heliovaara M, Viikari-Juntura E. Role of overweight and obesity in low back disorders among men: a longitudinal study with a life course approach. *BMJ Open.* 2015;5(8):e007805.

12. Jiang L, Tian W, Wang Y, et al. Body mass index and susceptibility to knee osteoarthritis: a systematic review and meta-analysis. *Joint Bone Spine.* 2012;79(3):291–297.

13. Jiang L, Rong J, Wang Y, et al. The relationship between body mass index and hip osteoarthritis: a systematic review and meta-analysis. *Joint Bone Spine.* 2011;78(2):150–155.

14. Yusuf E, Nelissen RG, Ioan-Facsinay A, et al. Association between weight or body mass index and hand osteoarthritis: a systematic review. *Ann Rheum Dis.* 2010;69(4):761–765.

15. Neumann L, Lerner E, Glazer Y, Bolotin A, Shefer A, Buskila D. A cross-sectional study of the relationship between body mass index and clinical characteristics, tenderness measures, quality of life, and physical functioning in fibromyalgia patients. *Clin Rheumatol.* 2008;27(12):1543–1547.

16. Okifuji A, Donaldson GW, Barck L, Fine PG. Relationship between fibromyalgia and obesity in pain, function, mood, and sleep. *J Pain.* 2010;11(12):1329–1337.

17. Mork PJ, Vasseljen O, Nilsen TI. Association between physical exercise, body mass index, and risk of fibromyalgia: longitudinal data from the Norwegian Nord-Trondelag Health Study. *Arthritis Care Res.* 2010;62(5):611–617.

18. Kim CH, Luedtke CA, Vincent A, Thompson JM, Oh TH. Association of body mass index with symptom severity and quality of life in patients with fibromyalgia. *Arthritis Care Res.* 2012;64(2):222–228.

19. Chai NC, Scher AI, Moghekar A, Bond DS, Peterlin BL. Obesity and headache: part I—a systematic review of the epidemiology of obesity and headache. *Headache.* 2014;54(2):219–234.

20. Runhaar J, Koes BW, Clockaerts S, Bierma-Zeinstra SM. A systematic review on changed biomechanics of lower extremities in obese individuals: a possible role in development of osteoarthritis. *Obes Rev.* 2011;12(12):1071–1082.

21. Chai NC, Bond DS, Moghekar A, Scher AI, Peterlin BL. Obesity and headache: Part II—potential mechanism and treatment considerations. *Headache.* 2014;54(3):459–471.

22. Christensen R, Bartels EM, Astrup A, Bliddal H. Effect of weight reduction in obese patients diagnosed with knee osteoarthritis: a systematic review and meta-analysis. *Ann Rheum Dis.* 2007;66(4):433–439.

23. Bliddal H, Leeds AR, Christensen R. Osteoarthritis, obesity and weight loss: evidence, hypotheses and horizons—a scoping review. *Obes Rev.* 2014;15(7):578–586.

24. Vincent HK, Heywood K, Connelly J, Hurley RW. Obesity and weight loss in the treatment and prevention of osteoarthritis. *PM&R.* 2012;4(5 Suppl.):S59–67.

25. Ursini F, Naty S, Grembiale RD. Fibromyalgia and obesity: the hidden link. *Rheumatol Int.* 2011;31(11):1403–1408.

26. Messier SP, Mihalko SL, Legault C, et al. Effects of intensive diet and exercise on knee joint loads, inflammation, and clinical outcomes among overweight and obese adults with knee osteoarthritis: the IDEA randomized clinical trial. *JAMA.* 2013;310(12):1263–1273.

27. Kerns RD, Sellinger J, Goodin BR. Psychological treatment of chronic pain. *Annu Rev Clin Psychol.* 2011;7:411–434.

28. Mauro M, Taylor V, Wharton S, Sharma AM. Barriers to obesity treatment. *Eur J Intern Med.* 2008;19(3):173–180.

29. Howarth D, Inman D, Lingard E, McCaskie A, Gerrand C. Barriers to weight loss in obese patients with knee osteoarthritis. *Ann R Coll Surg Engl.* 2010;92(4):338–340.

30. Wachholtz A, Binks M, Eisenson H, Kolotkin R, Suzuki A. Does pain predict interference with daily functioning and weight loss in an obese residential treatment-seeking population? *Int J Behav Med.* 2010;17(2):118–124.

31. Sellinger JJ, Clark EA, Shulman M, Rosenberger PH, Heapy AA, Kerns RD. The moderating effect of obesity on cognitive-behavioral pain treatment outcomes. *Pain Med.* 2010;11(9):1381–1390.

32. Janke EA, Kozak AT. "The more pain I have, the more I want to eat": obesity in the context of chronic pain. *Obesity.* 2012;20(10):2027–2034.

33. Teixeira PJ, Carraca EV, Marques MM, et al. Successful behavior change in obesity interventions in adults: a systematic review of self-regulation mediators. *BMC Med.* 2015;13:84.

34. Jensen MP, Nielson WR, Kerns RD. Toward the development of a motivational model of pain self-management. *J Pain.* 2003;4(9):477–492.

35. Webber KH, Tate DF, Ward DS, Bowling JM. Motivation and its relationship to adherence to self-monitoring and weight loss in a 16-week Internet behavioral weight loss intervention. *J Nutr Educ Behav.* 2010;42(3):161–167.

36. Dunkley AJ, Bodicoat DH, Greaves CJ, et al. Diabetes prevention in the real world: Effectiveness of pragmatic lifestyle interventions for the prevention of type 2 diabetes and of the impact of adherence to guideline recommendations: a systematic review and meta-analysis. *Diabetes Care.* 2014;37(4):922–933.

37. Johnston BC, Kanters S, Bandayrel K, et al. Comparison of weight loss among named diet programs in overweight and obese adults: a meta-analysis. *JAMA.* 2014;312(9):923–933.

38. Sacks FM, Bray GA, Carey VJ, et al. Comparison of weight-loss diets with different compositions of fat, protein, and carbohydrates. *N Engl J Med.* 2009;360(9):859–873.

39. Elfhag K, Rossner S. Who succeeds in maintaining weight loss? A conceptual review of factors associated with weight loss maintenance and weight regain. *Obes Rev.* 2005;6(1):67–85.

40. Franz MJ, VanWormer JJ, Crain AL, et al. Weight-loss outcomes: a systematic review and meta-analysis of weight-loss clinical trials with a minimum 1-year follow-up. *J Am Diet Assoc.* 2007;107(10):1755–1767.

41. Sanderson KB, Roditi D, George SZ, Atchison JW, Banou E, Robinson ME. Investigating patient expectations and treatment outcome in a chronic low back pain population. *J Pain Res.* 2012;5:15–22.

42. Fabricatore AN, Wadden TA, Womble LG, et al. The role of patients' expectations and goals in the behavioral and pharmacological treatment of obesity. *Int J Obes.* 2007;31(11):1739–1745.

43. Puhl RM, Heuer CA. The stigma of obesity: a review and update. *Obesity.* 2009;17(5):941–964.

44. Ockene JK, Schneider KL, Lemon SC, Ockene IS. Can we improve adherence to preventive therapies for cardiovascular health? *Circulation.* 2011;124(11): 1276–1282.

45. Fogelholm M. Physical activity, fitness and fatness: relations to mortality, morbidity and disease risk factors. A systematic review. *Obes Rev.* 2010;11(3):202–221.

46. Kratz AL, Molton IR, Jensen MP, Ehde DM, Nielson WR. Further evaluation of the Motivational Model of Pain Self-Management: coping with chronic pain in multiple sclerosis. *Ann Behav Med.* 2011;41(3):391–400.

47. Avena NM, Bocarsly ME, Hoebel BG, Gold MS. Overlaps in the nosology of substance abuse and overeating: the translational implications of "food addiction." *Curr Drug Abuse Rev.* 2011;4(3):133–139.

48. Volkow ND, Wang GJ, Tomasi D, Baler RD. Obesity and addiction: Neurobiological overlaps. *Obes Rev.* 2013;14(1):2–18.

49. Goldstone AP, Prechtl de Hernandez CG, Beaver JD, et al. Fasting biases brain reward systems towards high-calorie foods. *Eur J Neurosci.* 2009;30(8):1625–1635.

50. Jarcho JM, Mayer EA, Jiang ZK, Feier NA, London ED. Pain, affective symptoms, and cognitive deficits in patients with cerebral dopamine dysfunction. *Pain.* 2012;153(4):744–754.

51. Gandhi W, Becker S, Schweinhardt P. Pain increases motivational drive to obtain reward, but does not affect associated hedonic responses: a behavioural study in healthy volunteers. *Eur J Pain.* 2013;17(7):1093–1103.

52. Deckersbach T, Das SK, Urban LE, et al. Pilot randomized trial demonstrating reversal of obesity-related abnormalities in reward system responsivity to food cues with a behavioral intervention. *Nutr Diabetes.* 2014;4:e129.

53. Scholtz S, Miras AD, Chhina N, et al. Obese patients after gastric bypass surgery have lower brain-hedonic responses to food than after gastric banding. *Gut.* 2014;63(6):891–902.

54. Smith E, Hay P, Campbell L, Trollor JN. A review of the association between obesity and cognitive function across the lifespan: implications for novel approaches to prevention and treatment. *Obes Rev.* 2011;12(9):740–755.

55. Osika W, Montgomery SM, Longitudinal Birth Cohort Study. Physical control and coordination in childhood and adult obesity: Longitudinal Birth Cohort Study. *BMJ.* 2008;337:a699.

56. Wirt T, Schreiber A, Kesztyus D, Steinacker JM. Early life cognitive abilities and body weight: cross-sectional study of the association of inhibitory control, cognitive flexibility, and sustained attention with BMI percentiles in primary school children. *J Obes.* 2015;2015:534651.

57. Riggs N, Chou CP, Spruijt-Metz D, Pentz MA. Executive cognitive function as a correlate and predictor of child food intake and physical activity. *Child Neuropsychol.* 2010;16(3):279–292.

58. Appelhans BM, Woolf K, Pagoto SL, Schneider KL, Whited MC, Liebman R. Inhibiting food reward: delay discounting, food reward sensitivity, and palatable food intake in overweight and obese women. *Obesity.* 2011;19(11):2175–2182.

59. Nguyen JC, Killcross AS, Jenkins TA. Obesity and cognitive decline: role of inflammation and vascular changes. *Front Neurosci.* 2014;8:375.

60. Apkarian AV, Hashmi JA, Baliki MN. Pain and the brain: specificity and plasticity of the brain in clinical chronic pain. *Pain.* 2011;152(3 Suppl.):S49–64.

61. Moriarty O, McGuire BE, Finn DP. The effect of pain on cognitive function: a review of clinical and preclinical research. *Prog Neurobiol.* 2011;93(3):385–404.

62. Berryman C, Stanton TR, Jane Bowering K, Tabor A, McFarlane A, Lorimer Moseley G. Evidence for working memory deficits in chronic pain: a systematic review and meta-analysis. *Pain.* 2013;154(8):1181–1196.

63. Stilley CS, Bender CM, Dunbar-Jacob J, Sereika S, Ryan CM. The impact of cognitive function on medication management: three studies. *Health Psychol.* 2010;29(1):50–55.

64. Feil DG, Zhu CW, Sultzer DL. The relationship between cognitive impairment and diabetes self-management in a population-based community sample of older adults with Type 2 diabetes. *J Behav Med.* 2012;35(2):190–199.

65. Spitznagel MB, Garcia S, Miller LA, et al. Cognitive function predicts weight loss after bariatric surgery. *Surg Obes Relat Dis.* 2013;9(3):453–459.

66. Spitznagel MB, Alosco M, Galioto R, et al. The role of cognitive function in postoperative weight loss outcomes: 36-month follow-up. *Obes Surg.* 2014;24(7):1078–1084.

67. Galioto R, Gunstad J, Heinberg LJ, Spitznagel MB. Adherence and weight loss outcomes in bariatric surgery: does cognitive function play a role? *Obes Surg.* 2013;23(10):1703–1710.

68. Weber E, Blackstone K, Woods SP. Cognitive neurorehabilitation of HIV-associated neurocognitive disorders: a qualitative review and call to action. *Neuropsychol Rev.* 2013;23(1):81–98.

69. Skinner BF. *The Behavior of Organisms: An Experimental Analysis.* New York: D. Appleton-Century; 1938.

70. Appelhans BM, French SA, Pagoto SL, Sherwood NE. Managing temptation in obesity treatment: a neurobehavioral model of intervention strategies. *Appetite.* 2016;96:268–279.

71. Thorgeirsson T, Kawachi I. Behavioral economics: merging psychology and economics for lifestyle interventions. *Am J Prev Med.* 2013;44(2):185–189.

72. Roberto CA, Kawachi I. Use of psychology and behavioral economics to promote healthy eating. *Am J Prev Med.* 2014;47(6):832–837.

73. Gearhardt AN, Bragg MA, Pearl RL, Schvey NA, Roberto CA, Brownell KD. Obesity and public policy. *Annu Rev Clin Psychol.* 2012;8:405–430.

74. Ouwehand C, Papies EK. Eat it or beat it. The differential effects of food temptations on overweight and normal-weight restrained eaters. *Appetite.* 2010;55(1):56–60.

75. Buehler R, Griffin D, Ross M. Exploring the "planning fallacy": why pople underestimate their task completion times. *J Pers Soc Psychol.* 1994;67(3):366–381.

76. Wansink B. From mindless eating to mindlessly eating better. *Physiol Behav.* 2010;100(5):454–463.

77. Sykes-Muskett BJ, Prestwich A, Lawton RJ, Armitage CJ. The utility of monetary contingency contracts for weight loss: a systematic review and meta-analysis. *Health Psychol Rev.* 2015;9(4):434–451.

78. Purnell JQ, Gernes R, Stein R, Sherraden MS, Knoblock-Hahn A. A systematic review of financial incentives for dietary behavior change. *J Acad Nutr Diet.* 2014;114(7):1023–1035.

79. Mitchell MS, Goodman JM, Alter DA, et al. Financial incentives for exercise adherence in adults: systematic review and meta-analysis. *Am J Prev Med.* 2013;45(5):658–667.

80. Bandura A. *Self-Efficacy: The Exercise of Control.* New York: Freeman; 1997.

81. Szabo-Reed AN, Lee J, Ptomey L, et al. Longitudinal weight loss patterns and their behavioral and demographic associations. *Ann Behav Med.* 2016;50(1):147–156.

82. Burke LE, Ewing LJ, Ye L, et al. The SELF trial: a self-efficacy-based behavioral intervention trial for weight loss maintenance. *Obesity.* 2015;23(11):2175–2182.

83. Pincus T, Smeets RJ, Simmonds MJ, Sullivan MJ. The fear avoidance model disentangled: improving the clinical utility of the fear avoidance model. *Clin J Pain.* 2010;26(9):739–746.

84. Leeuw M, Goossens ME, Linton SJ, Crombez G, Boersma K, Vlaeyen JW. The fear-avoidance model of musculoskeletal pain: current state of scientific evidence. *J Behav Med.* 2007;30(1):77–94.

85. Stewart SH, Asmundson GJ. Anxiety sensitivity and its impact on pain experiences and conditions: a state of the art. *Cogn Behav Ther.* 2006;35(4):185–188.

86. Somers TJ, Keefe FJ, Carson JW, Pells JJ, Lacaille L. Pain catastrophizing in borderline morbidly obese and morbidly obese individuals with osteoarthritic knee pain. *Pain Res Manag.* 2008;13(5):401–406.

87. Janke EA, Jones E, Hopkins CM, Ruggieri M, Hruska A. Catastrophizing and anxiety sensitivity mediate the relationship between persistent pain and emotional eating. *Appetite.* 2016;103:64–71.

88. Shelby RA, Somers TJ, Keefe FJ, Pells JJ, Dixon KE, Blumenthal JA. Domain specific self-efficacy mediates the impact of pain catastrophizing on pain and disability in overweight and obese osteoarthritis patients. *J Pain.* 2008;9(10):912–919.

89. Smits JA, Tart CD, Presnell K, Rosenfield D, Otto MW. Identifying potential barriers to physical activity adherence: anxiety sensitivity and body mass as predictors of fear during exercise. *Cogn Behav Ther.* 2010;39(1):28–36.

90. Vincent HK, Omli MR, Day T, Hodges M, Vincent KR, George SZ. Fear of movement, quality of life, and self-reported disability in obese patients with chronic lumbar pain. *Pain Med.* 2011;12(1):154–164.
91. Zale EL, Lange KL, Fields SA, Ditre JW. The relation between pain-related fear and disability: a meta-analysis. *J Pain.* 2013;14(10):1019–1030.
92. Wertli MM, Rasmussen-Barr E, Held U, Weiser S, Bachmann LM, Brunner F. Fear-avoidance beliefs—a moderator of treatment efficacy in patients with low back pain: a systematic review. *Spine J.* 2014;14(11):2658–2678.
93. Vincent HK, Adams MC, Vincent KR, Hurley RW. Musculoskeletal pain, fear avoidance behaviors, and functional decline in obesity: potential interventions to manage pain and maintain function. *Reg Anesth Pain Med.* 2013;38(6):481–491.
94. Christakis NA, Fowler JH. The spread of obesity in a large social network over 32 years. *N Engl J Med.* 2007;357(4):370–379.
95. Leahey TM, Doyle CY, Xu X, Bihuniak J, Wing RR. Social networks and social norms are associated with obesity treatment outcomes. *Obesity.* 2015;23(8):1550–1554.
96. Wing RR, Leahey T, Jeffery R, et al. Do weight loss and adherence cluster within behavioral treatment groups? *Obesity.* 2014;22(3):638–644.
97. Leroux JS, Moore S, Dube L. Beyond the "I" in the obesity epidemic: a review of social relational and network interventions on obesity. *J Obes.* 2013:348249.
98. Litt MD, Kadden RM, Kabela-Cormier E, Petry NM. Changing network support for drinking: network support project 2-year follow-up. *J Consult Clin Psychol.* 2009;77(2):229–242.
99. Li JS, Barnett TA, Goodman E, et al. Approaches to the prevention and management of childhood obesity: the role of social networks and the use of social media and related electronic technologies: a scientific statement from the American Heart Association. *Circulation.* 2013;127(2):260–267.
100. Ludwig J, Duncan GJ, Gennetian LA, et al. Neighborhood effects on the long-term well-being of low-income adults. *Science.* 2012;337(6101):1505–1510.
101. Drewnowski A, Moudon AV, Jiao J, Aggarwal A, Charreire H, Chaix B. Food environment and socioeconomic status influence obesity rates in Seattle and in Paris. *Int J Obes.* 2014;38(2):306–314.
102. Grow HM, Cook AJ, Arterburn DE, Saelens BE, Drewnowski A, Lozano P. Child obesity associated with social disadvantage of children's neighborhoods. *Soc Sci Med.* 2010;71(3):584–591.
103. Saelens BE, Sallis JF, Frank LD, et al. Obesogenic neighborhood environments, child and parent obesity: the Neighborhood Impact on Kids study. *Am J Prev Med.* 2012;42(5):e57–64.
104. Carroll-Scott A, Gilstad-Hayden K, Rosenthal L, et al. Disentangling neighborhood contextual associations with child body mass index, diet, and physical activity: the role of built, socioeconomic, and social environments. *Soc Sci Med.* 2013;95:106–114.
105. Auchincloss AH, Mujahid MS, Shen M, Michos ED, Whitt-Glover MC, Diez Roux AV. Neighborhood health-promoting resources and obesity risk (the multi-ethnic study of atherosclerosis). *Obesity.* 2013;21(3):621–628.
106. Mayne SL, Auchincloss AH, Michael YL. Impact of policy and built environment changes on obesity-related outcomes: a systematic review of naturally occurring experiments. *Obes Rev.* 2015;16(5):362–375.
107. Department of Veterans Affairs. *VA/DoD Clinical Practice Guideline for Screening and Management of Overweight and Obesity.* Office of Quality and Performance

publication 10Q-CPG/Obesity-06. Washington, DC: Department of Veterans Affairs; 2014.

108. National Institute for Health and Care Excellence. *Obesity: Identification, Assessment and Management.* Clinical Guideline 189. November 27, 2014; https://www.nice.org.uk/guidance/cg189. Accessed February 1, 2016.

109. Woolf AD, Breedveld F, Kvien TK. Controlling the obesity epidemic is important for maintaining musculoskeletal health. *Ann Rheum Dis.* 2006;65(11): 1401–1402.

110. Hochberg MC, Altman RD, April KT, et al. American College of Rheumatology 2012 recommendations for the use of nonpharmacologic and pharmacologic therapies in osteoarthritis of the hand, hip, and knee. *Arthritis Care Res.* 2012;64(4):465–474.

111. EBaJHS. European Action Towards Better Musculoskeletal Health: A Public Health Strategy to Reduce the Burden of Musculoskeletal Conditions. 2005;1. National Institute for Health and Care Excellence. *Obesity: Identification, Assessment and Management.* Clinical Guideline 189. November 27, 2014; https://www.nice.org.uk/guidance/cg189. Accessed February 1, 2016.

112. Harris JA, Benedict FG. A biometric study of human basal metabolism. *Proc Natl Acad Sci USA.* 1918;4(12):370–373.

113. Garber CE, Blissmer B, Deschenes MR, et al. American College of Sports Medicine position stand. Quantity and quality of exercise for developing and maintaining cardiorespiratory, musculoskeletal, and neuromotor fitness in apparently healthy adults: guidance for prescribing exercise. *Med Sci Sports Exerc.* 2011;43(7):1334–1359.

114. Janke EA, Ramirez ML, Haltzman B, Fritz M, Kozak AT. Patient's experience with comorbidity management in primary care: a qualitative study of comorbid pain and obesity. *Prim Health Care Res Dev.* 2016;17(1):33–41.

115. Dorflinger L, Kerns RD, Auerbach SM. Providers' roles in enhancing patients' adherence to pain self management. *Transl Behav Med.* 2013;3(1):39–46.

116. Durant NH, Bartman B, Person SD, Collins F, Austin SB. Patient–provider communication about the health effects of obesity. *Patient Educ Couns.* 2009;75(1):53–57.

117. Upshur CC, Bacigalupe G, Luckmann R. "They don't want anything to do with you": patient views of primary care management of chronic pain. *Pain Med.* 2010;11(12):1791–1798.

118. Malterud K, Ulriksen K. Obesity, stigma, and responsibility in health care: a synthesis of qualitative studies. *Int J Qual Stud Health Well-Being.* 2011;6(4).

119. Bordin ES. The generalizability of the psychoanalytic concept of working alliance. *Psychother Theory Res Pract.* 1979;16(3):252–260.

120. Wampold BE. Outcomes of individual counseling and psychotherapy: empirical evidence addressing two fundamental questions. In: Brown SD, Lent RW, eds. *Handbook of Counseling Psychology,* 3rd ed. Hoboken, NJ: John Wiley; 2000:711–739.

121. Mead N, Bower P. Patient-centred consultations and outcomes in primary care: a review of the literature. *Patient Educ Couns.* 2002;48(1):51–61.

122. Fuertes JN, Mislowack A, Bennett J, et al. The physician–patient working alliance. *Patient Educ Couns.* 2007;66(1):29–36.

123. Fuertes JN, Boylan LS, Fontanella JA. Behavioral indices in medical care outcome: the working alliance, adherence, and related factors. *J Gen Intern Med.* 2009;24(1):80–85.

124. Street RL Jr, De Haes HC. Designing a curriculum for communication skills training from a theory and evidence-based perspective. *Patient Educ Couns.* 2013;93(1):27–33.

125. Vong SK, Cheing GL, Chan F, So EM, Chan CC. Motivational enhancement therapy in addition to physical therapy improves motivational factors and treatment outcomes in people with low back pain: a randomized controlled trial. *Arch Phys Med Rehabil.* 2011;92(2):176–183.

126. Alperstein D, Sharpe L. The efficacy of motivational interviewing in adults with chronic pain: a meta-analysis and systematic review. *J Pain.* 2016;17(4):393–403.

127. Armstrong MJ, Mottershead TA, Ronksley PE, Sigal RJ, Campbell TS, Hemmelgarn BR. Motivational interviewing to improve weight loss in overweight and/or obese patients: a systematic review and meta-analysis of randomized controlled trials. *Obes Rev.* Sep 2011;12(9):709–723.

128. Miller WR, Rose GS. Toward a theory of motivational interviewing. *Am Psychol.* 2009;64(6):527–537.

129. Phelan SM, Burgess DJ, Yeazel MW, Hellerstedt WL, Griffin JM, van Ryn M. Impact of weight bias and stigma on quality of care and outcomes for patients with obesity. *Obes Rev.* 2015;16(4):319–326.

130. Teachman BA, Brownell KD. Implicit anti-fat bias among health professionals: is anyone immune? *Int J Obes Relat Metab Disord.* 2001;25(10):1525–1531.

131. Bacon JG, Scheltema KE, Robinson BE. Fat Phobia Scale revisited: the short form. *Int J Obes Relat Metab Disord.* 2001;25(2):252–257.

132. Morrison TG, O'Connor WE. Psychometric properties of a scale measuring negative attitudes toward overweight individuals. *J Soc Psychol.* 1999;139(4):436–445.

133. Allison DB, Basile VC, Yuker HE. The measurement of attitudes toward and beliefs about obese persons. *Int J Eat Disord.* 1991;10(5):599–607.

134. Kushner RF. *Roadmaps for Clinical Practice: Case Studies in Disease Prevention and Health Promotion-Assessment and Management of Adult Obesity: A Primer for physicians.* Chicago: American Medical Association; 2003.

135. Tylka TL, Annunziato RA, Burgard D, et al. The weight-inclusive versus weight-normative approach to health: evaluating the evidence for prioritizing well-being over weight loss. *J Obes.* 2014;2014:983495.

136. Puhl R, Peterson JL, Luedicke J. Motivating or stigmatizing? Public perceptions of weight-related language used by health providers. *Int J Obes.* 2013;37(4):612–619.

137. Rose SA, Poynter PS, Anderson JW, Noar SM, Conigliaro J. Physician weight loss advice and patient weight loss behavior change: a literature review and meta-analysis of survey data. *Int J Obes.* 2013;37(1):118–128.

138. Rueda-Clausen CF, Benterud E, Bond T, Olszowka R, Vallis MT, Sharma AM. Effect of implementing the 5As of obesity management framework on provider-patient interactions in primary care. *Clin Obes.* 2014;4(1):39–44.

139. Jay M, Gillespie C, Schlair S, Sherman S, Kalet A. Physicians' use of the 5As in counseling obese patients: is the quality of counseling associated with patients' motivation and intention to lose weight? *BMC Health Serv Res.* 2010;10:159.

140. Dalle Grave R, Calugi S, Molinari E, et al. Weight loss expectations in obese patients and treatment attrition: an observational multicenter study. *Obes Res.* 2005;13(11):1961–1969.

141. Prochaska JO, DiClemente CC. *The Transtheoretical Approach: Crossing Traditional Boundaries of Therapy.* Homewood, IL: Dow Jones-Irwin; 1984.

142. Prochaska JO, DiClemente CC, Norcross JC. In search of how people change. applications to addictive behaviors. *Am Psychol.* 1992;47(9):1102–1114.

143. Andres A, Saldana C, Gomez-Benito J. Establishing the stages and processes of change for weight loss by consensus of experts. *Obesity.* 2009;17(9):1717–1723.

144. Logue E, Sutton K, Jarjoura D, Smucker W. Obesity management in primary care: assessment of readiness to change among 284 family practice patients. *J Am Board Fam Pract.* 2000;13(3):164–171.

145. Luppino FS, de Wit LM, Bouvy PF, et al. Overweight, obesity, and depression: a systematic review and meta-analysis of longitudinal studies. *Arch Gen Psychiatry.* 2010;67(3):220–229.

146. Burke AL, Mathias JL, Denson LA. Psychological functioning of people living with chronic pain: a meta-analytic review. *Br J Clin Psychol.* 2015;54(3):345–360.

147. Tietjen GE, Peterlin BL, Brandes JL, et al. Depression and anxiety: effect on the migraine-obesity relationship. *Headache.* 2007;47(6):866–875.

148. Konttinen H, Mannisto S, Sarlio-Lahteenkorva S, Silventoinen K, Haukkala A. Emotional eating, depressive symptoms and self-reported food consumption. A population-based study. *Appetite.* 2010;54(3):473–479.

149. Ball K, Burton NW, Brown WJ. A prospective study of overweight, physical activity, and depressive symptoms in young women. *Obesity.* 2009;17(1):66–71.

150. Messier SP. Diet and exercise for obese adults with knee osteoarthritis. *Clin Geriatr Med.* 2010;26(3):461–477.

151. Messier SP, Loeser RF, Miller GD, et al. Exercise and dietary weight loss in overweight and obese older adults with knee osteoarthritis: the Arthritis, Diet, and Activity Promotion Trial. *Arthritis Rheum.* 2004;50(5):1501–1510.

152. Wadden TA, Webb VL, Moran CH, Bailer BA. Lifestyle modification for obesity: new developments in diet, physical activity, and behavior therapy. *Circulation.* 2012;125(9):1157–1170.

153. Bodenheimer T, Handley MA. Goal-setting for behavior change in primary care: an exploration and status report. *Patient Educ Couns.* 2009;76(2):174–180.

154. Durant NH, Joseph RP, Affuso OH, Dutton GR, Robertson HT, Allison DB. Empirical evidence does not support an association between less ambitious pre-treatment goals and better treatment outcomes: a meta-analysis. *Obes Rev.* 2013;14(7):532–540.

155. Freund AM, Hennecke M. Changing eating behaviour vs. losing weight: the role of goal focus for weight loss in overweight women. *Psychol Health.* 2012;27 Suppl 2:25–42.

156. Raaijmakers LC, Pouwels S, Berghuis KA, Nienhuijs SW. Technology-based interventions in the treatment of overweight and obesity: a systematic review. *Appetite.* Dec 2015;95:138–151.

157. Boudreaux ED, Waring ME, Hayes RB, Sadasivam RS, Mullen S, Pagoto S. Evaluating and selecting mobile health apps: strategies for healthcare providers and healthcare organizations. *Transl Behav Med.* 2014;4(4):363–371.

158. Bond DS, Buse DC, Lipton RB, et al. Clinical pain catastrophizing in women with migraine and obesity. *Headache.* 2015;55(7):923–933.

159. Darnall BD, Sturgeon JA, Kao MC, Hah JM, Mackey SC. From catastrophizing to recovery: a pilot study of a single-session treatment for pain catastrophizing. *J Pain Res.* 2014;7:219–226.

160. Somers TJ, Wren AA, Blumenthal JA, Caldwell D, Huffman KM, Keefe FJ. Pain, physical functioning, and overeating in obese rheumatoid arthritis patients: do thoughts about pain and eating matter? *J Clin Rheumatol.* 2014;20(5):244–250.

161. Sallis JF, Pinski RB, Grossman RM, Patterson TL, Nader PR. The development of self-efficacy scales for health-related diet and exercise behaviors. *Health Educ Res.* 1988;3(3):283–292.

162. Akkaya N, Akkaya S, Atalay NS, Balci CS, Sahin F. Relationship between the body image and level of pain, functional status, severity of depression, and quality of life in patients with fibromyalgia syndrome. *Clin Rheumatol.* 2012;31(6):983–988.

163. Robinson AH, Adler S, Stevens HB, Darcy AM, Morton JM, Safer DL. What variables are associated with successful weight loss outcomes for bariatric surgery after 1 year? *Surg Obes Relat Dis.* 2014;10(4):697–704.

164. Roberts MH, Klatzkin RR, Mechlin B. Social support attenuates physiological stress responses and experimental pain sensitivity to cold pressor pain. *Ann Behav Med.* 2015;49(4):557–569.

165. Wadden TA, Butryn ML, Hong PS, Tsai AG. Behavioral treatment of obesity in patients encountered in primary care settings: a systematic review. *JAMA.* 2014;312(17):1779–1791.

166. Nelson AE, Allen KD, Golightly YM, Goode AP, Jordan JM. A systematic review of recommendations and guidelines for the management of osteoarthritis: the chronic osteoarthritis management initiative of the U.S. bone and joint initiative. *Semin Arthritis Rheum.* 2014;43(6):701–712.

167. Ambrose KR, Golightly YM. Physical exercise as non-pharmacological treatment of chronic pain: why and when. *Best Pract Res Clin Rheumatol.* 2015;29(1):120–130.

168. Bennell KL, Hinman RS. A review of the clinical evidence for exercise in osteoarthritis of the hip and knee. *J Sci Med Sport.* 2011;14(1):4–9.

169. Golightly YM, Allen KD, Caine DJ. A comprehensive review of the effectiveness of different exercise programs for patients with osteoarthritis. *Phys Sportsmed.* 2012;40(4):52–65.

170. Roddy E, Zhang W, Doherty M, et al. Evidence-based recommendations for the role of exercise in the management of osteoarthritis of the hip or knee—the MOVE consensus. *Rheumatology.* 2005;44(1):67–73.

171. Bennell KL, Dobson F, Hinman RS. Exercise in osteoarthritis: moving from prescription to adherence. *Best Pract Res Clin Rheumatol.* 2014;28(1):93–117.

172. Song J, Hochberg MC, Chang RW, et al. Racial and ethnic differences in physical activity guidelines attainment among people at high risk of or having knee osteoarthritis. *Arthritis Care Res.* 2013;65(2):195–202.

173. Jones KD, Adams D, Winters-Stone K, Burckhardt CS. A comprehensive review of 46 exercise treatment studies in fibromyalgia (1988–2005). *Health Qual Life Outcomes.* 2006;4:67.

174. Barker AL, Talevski J, Morello RT, Brand CA, Rahmann AE, Urquhart DM. Effectiveness of aquatic exercise for musculoskeletal conditions: a meta-analysis. *Arch Phys Med Rehabil.* 2014;95(9):1776–1786.

175. Uthman OA, van der Windt DA, Jordan JL, et al. Exercise for lower limb osteoarthritis: systematic review incorporating trial sequential analysis and network meta-analysis. *BMJ.* 2013;347:f5555.

176. Searle A, Spink M, Ho A, Chuter V. Exercise interventions for the treatment of chronic low back pain: a systematic review and meta-analysis of randomised controlled trials. *Clin Rehabil.* 2015;29(12):1155–1167.

177. Zhang W, Nuki G, Moskowitz RW, et al. OARSI recommendations for the management of hip and knee osteoarthritis: part III: changes in evidence following

systematic cumulative update of research published through January 2009. *Osteoarthritis Cartilage.* 2010;18(4):476–499.

178. Fransen M, McConnell S, Harmer AR, Van der Esch M, Simic M, Bennell KL. Exercise for osteoarthritis of the knee. *Cochrane Database Syst Rev.* 2015;1:CD004376.

179. Wallis JA, Taylor NF. Pre-operative interventions (non-surgical and non-pharmacological) for patients with hip or knee osteoarthritis awaiting joint replacement surgery—a systematic review and meta-analysis. *Osteoarthritis Cartilage.* 2011;19(12):1381–1395.

180. Steffens D, Maher CG, Pereira LS, et al. Prevention of low back pain: a systematic review and meta-analysis. *JAMA Intern Med.* 2016:1–10.

181. Pisters MF, Veenhof C, van Meeteren NL, et al. Long-term effectiveness of exercise therapy in patients with osteoarthritis of the hip or knee: a systematic review. *Arthritis Rheum.* 2007;57(7):1245–1253.

182. Pisters MF, Veenhof C, Schellevis FG, Twisk JW, Dekker J, De Bakker DH. Exercise adherence improving long-term patient outcome in patients with osteoarthritis of the hip and/or knee. *Arthritis Care Res.* 2010;62(8):1087–1094.

183. Fransen M, McConnell S. Exercise for osteoarthritis of the knee. *Cochrane Database Syst Rev.* 2008(4):CD004376.

184. Ravaud P, Giraudeau B, Logeart I, et al. Management of osteoarthritis (OA) with an unsupervised home based exercise programme and/or patient administered assessment tools: a cluster randomised controlled trial with a 2×2 factorial design. *Ann Rheum Dis.* 2004;63(6):703–708.

185. Li LC, Sayre EC, Kopec JA, Esdaile JM, Bar S, Cibere J. Quality of nonpharmacological care in the community for people with knee and hip osteoarthritis. *J Rheumatol.* 2011;38(10):2230–2237.

186. Brand CA, Ackerman IN, Bohensky MA, Bennell KL. Chronic disease management: a review of current performance across quality of care domains and opportunities for improving osteoarthritis care. *Rheum Dis Clin North Am.* 2013;39(1):123–143.

187. Austin S, Qu H, Shewchuk RM. Health care providers' recommendations for physical activity and adherence to physical activity guidelines among adults with arthritis. *Prev Chronic Dis.* 2013;10:E182.

188. Meneses SR, Goode AP, Nelson AE, et al. Clinical algorithms to aid osteoarthritis guideline dissemination. *Osteoarthritis Cartilage.* 2016;24(9):1487–1499.

189. Lobelo F, Stoutenberg M, Hutber A. The Exercise is Medicine Global Health Initiative: a 2014 update. *Br J Sports Med.* 2014;48(22):1627–1633.

190. Marks R. Knee osteoarthritis and exercise adherence: a review. *Curr Aging Sci.* 2012;5(1):72–83.

191. Petursdottir U, Arnadottir SA, Halldorsdottir S. Facilitators and barriers to exercising among people with osteoarthritis: a phenomenological study. *Phys Ther.* 2010;90(7):1014–1025.

192. Garver MJ, Focht BC, Taylor SJ. Integrating lifestyle approaches into osteoarthritis care. *J Multidiscip Healthc.* 2015;8:409–418.

193. Gay C, Chabaud A, Guilley E, Coudeyre E. Educating patients about the benefits of physical activity and exercise for their hip and knee osteoarthritis: systematic literature review. *Ann Phys Rehabil Med.* 2016;59(3):174–183.

CHAPTER 6

໑ఌ

Biopsychosocial Approach to Improving Treatment Adherence in Chronic Pain

MARTIN D. CHEATLE AND LARA DHINGRA

INTRODUCTION

Approximately 30% of the American population experiences recurrent or chronic pain.[1,2] Individuals with chronic pain can suffer greatly, but the disease of pain also affects family members and has enormous economic and societal consequences. For example, it has been estimated that between $560 billion and $600 billion is expended yearly on chronic pain.[3] To put this in perspective, costs associated with chronic pain far exceed what is expended on heart disease. Pain that is persistent often has complex etiologies, and patients present with multiple medical and psychological comorbidities. While a linear approach of symptoms leading to a diagnosis that determines a discreet treatment course has served the field of medicine well for a number of disease states, it has not been effective or efficacious for chronic pain.[4] Currently, most pain care models are either unimodal (spinal injections, radiofrequency ablations, spinal cord stimulation) or multimodal (interventional and pharmacotherapy), although evidence-based outcomes of long-term efficacy for these models are lacking.[5] There is strong evidence that a multimodal approach within an interdisciplinary, biopsychosocial framework is the most effective, clinically and economically, in managing patients with chronic pain.[6-8] A biopsychosocial program for chronic pain typically includes the appropriate use of pharmacotherapies that target pain, sleep, and mood disturbance; cognitive behavioral therapy (CBT); dietary change and weight management; restorative exercise; and enhanced social support.[9] While each of these components is efficacious in improving pain, function, and mood, barriers in access to care and adherence to the treatment regimen remains common. Other chapters in this book address theory-based interventions for improving treatment adherence in chronic pain, appropriate use and monitoring of medications, exercise, and nutrition/weight loss. This chapter focuses on the delivery of psychological interventions for pain populations, with an emphasis on the use of specific strategies to enhance adherence to psychological and pharmacologic interventions in chronic pain management.

Adherence Versus Nonadherence

Most research on adherence and nonadherence has been devoted to medication use in varied chronic illnesses (diabetes, hypertension, cancer, and HIV). However, adherence also is critical for a number of health behavior change interventions that have a significant impact on healthcare outcomes. These behaviors include smoking cessation, physical activity, dietary change, and adaptive coping with chronic illness. The construct of adherence is often used interchangeably with that of compliance. The World Health Organization defined adherence to long-term therapy as "The extent which a person's behavior—taking medication, following a diet, and/or executing lifestyle changes—corresponds with agreed recommendations from a healthcare provider (HCP)."[10] This definition emphasizes a collaborative relationship between the HCP and the patient, emphasizing effective communication between the patient and the HCP to maximize the probability of a positive and meaningful outcome from a therapeutic intervention. Compliance deemphasizes this collaborative approach and suggests that the communication style is that of the HCP instructing or preaching to the patient, and the patient's agreement with the prescribed intervention is neither sought nor relevant.

The HCP–Patient Relationship

The patient, though conscious that his condition is perilous, may recover his health simply through his contentment with the goodness of the physician.

Hippocrates

A collaborative relationship between the patient and the HCP is critical to improving treatment adherence and promotes improved patient satisfaction, which is increasingly important for outcome-based reimbursement in the changing healthcare system. For example, Farin et al.[11] examined the HCP–patient relationship among 686 patients with chronic low back pain as a predictor of treatment outcome after a rehabilitation program. The researchers assessed patient–physician relationship factors, including satisfaction with care, trust in the physician, and patient participation. They discovered that, after adjusting for sociodemographic, medical, and psychological factors, the patient–physician relationship was significantly associated with the outcomes of treatment (pain, disability, quality of life, and others). This effect was more robust at six months following rehabilitation completion. Similarly, the patient's perception of actively participating in medical decision-making was also associated with improved quality of life in women with breast cancer completing a rehabilitation program.[12] Conversely, a systematic review of determinants of medication nonadherence in patients with chronic pain revealed that an unsatisfactory HCP–patient relationship was a robust predictor of medication nonadherence.[13]

Studies suggest that establishing a HCP–patient relationship that facilitates patient engagement, shared decision-making, and effective communication through which a patient perceives that he or she is listened to and respected can lead to improved treatment adherence, enhancing both quality of life and patient satisfaction.

ASSESSMENT OF ADHERENCE BEHAVIOR

The assessment of adherence behaviors and the factors that can influence them is critical to optimizing pain management. The assessment of adherence should include a comprehensive history and clinical interview with the patient that includes the assessment of known risk factors for nonadherence and clinical, behavioral, and biometric measures.

Clinical Interview/Risk Assessment

An initial comprehensive clinical interview is essential in evaluating potential factors that can lead to treatment nonadherence. These factors include motivation and readiness for behavior change and the assessment of risk factors for nonadherence.

Motivation and Readiness for Change

Prior to implementing any treatment intervention, whether it is pharmacotherapy, rehabilitation, or psychological strategies to improve pain coping, assessing the patient's motivation to engage in behavior change is critical. The classic model by Prochaski and DeClemente[14] provides an empirically derived framework for classifying motivational level for behavior change. The authors suggested that there were five steps of change: (1) *precontemplation*—the individual has no intention to change a behavior and is not conscious of the need to change a behavior (e.g., has not considered smoking cessation or the long-term deleterious effects of smoking); (2) *contemplative*—the individual develops an awareness of a need to change a behavior (has developed a persistent cough, concerns raised by a significant other); (3) *preparation*—the individual begins preparing to take action within the next 30 days (e.g., obtains information regarding smoking cessation from the American Cancer Society, discusses his or her intent to quit smoking with a primary care physician, and obtains a prescription for a smoking cessation medication); (4) *action*—the individual implements steps to modify a particular behavior or environment (e.g., fills the prescription, enacts the behavioral steps acquired in the preparation phase to reduce and eventually discontinue smoking); and (5) *maintenance*—the individual consistently engages in the new healthy behaviors until they become solidified and second-nature.

Typically, many patients present to a HCP either at the precontemplative or contemplative stage; however, the HCP is most likely at the action stage (writing a prescription for physical therapy, pharmacotherapy, etc.). It is important to assess the patient's motivational drives and stage of readiness to change and begin prompting the patient from precontemplative to contemplative, to preparing for action, and, finally, to the maintenance stage. Supporting the patient's transitions from one stage to another involves increasing the relevance of the behavior change by personalizing the benefits and offering nonjudgmental education and heightened awareness about the unhealthy versus healthy behaviors and long-term consequences. For example, for a patient rooted in the precontemplative stage; engendering the individual's sense of self-empowerment, which is typically harnessed in the contemplation stage, and then providing specific behavior change strategies during the action/maintenance stage can strengthen coping skills and facilitate movement. When there is a mismatch between the patient and the HCP regarding these stages, this tends to lead to frustration for both parties and can undermine adherence.

Assessing Risk Factors for Nonadherence to Pain Interventions

There are a number of risk factors, including psychiatric and medical comorbidities, and situational factors that may undermine adherence to pain interventions. These problems include depression, anxiety, sleep disturbance, substance misuse, and socioeconomic factors (see Figure 6.1). It is imperative to assess for the presence of these potential risk factors that can diminish the efficacy of a well-designed treatment program and lead to potential negative consequences, including increased anxiety and depression, emergency room visits, and personal and family distress. Assessment may provide the HCP with the opportunity to preemptively manage these factors to improve adherence.

Depression and anxiety

It is well documented that depression and anxiety can promote nonadherence to therapeutic interventions in a number of medical conditions such as hypertension,[15] chronic obstructive pulmonary disease,[16] HIV,[17] and rheumatoid arthritis.[18] There are a number of well-validated and reliable assessment tools for depression (e.g., the Patient Health Questionnaire-9[19] and the Zung Self-Rating Depression Scale[20]) and anxiety (e.g., the Beck Anxiety Inventory[21]) and tools that measure both depression and anxiety

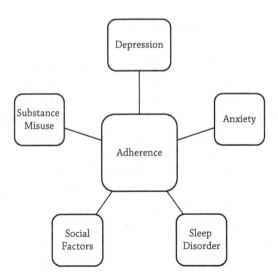

Figure 6.1. Risk factors for nonadherence.

(e.g., the Hospital Anxiety and Depression Scale[22]) in the general population. An expert consensus panel was convened to evaluate measuring emotional functioning in chronic pain[23] and recommended the use of the Beck
Depression Inventory[24] and the Profile of Mood States.[25]

Sleep disturbance

Between 50% and 80% of patients with chronic pain report moderate sleep
disturbance.[26,27] It has been well established that pain and sleep are bidirectional, with pain leading to sleep disturbance and sleep causing increased
pain via reduction in pain tolerance[28] and release of proinflammatory cyto-
kines.[29] Last, it has been demonstrated that sleep deprivation not only
leads to increased pain but also fatigue, stress, depression, and disability,
all of which can erode adherence.[30,31] Standard measures of sleep disturbance include polysomnography, self-report measures, and, more recently,
actigraphy. Self-report measures are most commonly employed, as they
are inexpensive and easy to complete and interpret. There are a number of
sleep assessment scales that measure varied dimensions of sleep from sleep
quality to postsleep evaluation to sleep onset. Post-sleep evaluation (e.g.,
Wolff's morning questions[32]) and sleep quality (Pittsburgh Sleep Quality
Questionnaire[33]) are the most widely used in clinical practice. Moul et al.[34]
provide a critical review of the major sleep measurement instruments.

Socioeconomic factors

A thorough history and clinical interview should include assessing specific socioeconomic factors that may directly affect adherence to prescribed therapies. For example, a recent systematic review[35] evaluated the
relationship of various social determinants of health and adherence and
motivation to complete programs of cardiac and cancer rehabilitation. The
results showed the most frequent social determinants of health factors
that influenced attendance and motivation were social support, transportation, employment status, income, housing, and food security. The clinician should be cognizant of these factors and not compromise patients'
success, for instance, by prescribing physical therapy on a three times per
week basis when the patient has limited access to transportation or cannot
afford co-pays. This will ultimately erode the HCP–patient relationship and
undermine adherence. Instead, options for self-management and a home
exercise program may be more cost-effective and achievable.

Substance misuse

Undetected substance misuse or abuse of medically prescribed opioids and benzodiazepines can reduce adherence and contribute to mood and sleep disorders. Assessing for substance misuse involves drug monitoring, careful physical examination (mild tremor, tender/enlarged liver, labile blood pressure), laboratory studies (elevated liver enzymes), and the use of validated assessment tools. Typical assessment tools comprise three categories: (a) prescreening tools when a patient is being considered for opioid therapy (e.g., the Opioid Risk Tool,[36] Screener and Opioid Assessment for Patients with Pain,[37] Diagnosis, Intractability, Risk, Efficacy,[38] and Drug Abuse Screening Test[39]); (b) monitoring tools for patients who are receiving long-term opioid therapy (e.g., the Pain Assessment and Documentation Tool[40] and the Current Opioid Misuse Measure[41]); and (c) generic tools for monitoring alcohol and/or illicit drug use (e.g., the Cut down, Annoyed, Guilty, Eye-opener tool Adjusted to include Drugs [CAGE-AID][42]). While the opioid misuse measurement instruments have specific methodological limitations, such as generalizability (most were developed using patients treated in pain settings) and issues inherent with self-report measures (e.g., response bias),[43] they can have merit if used as one component of a comprehensive risk assessment approach.

Clinical, Behavioral, and Biometric Measures of Adherence

A number of approaches have been developed to assess adherence or nonadherence to pharmacologic and behavioral interventions. These include the use of patient self-report, behaviors, and improvement in objective clinical outcomes (e.g., blood pressure recordings, HbA_{1c}, etc.) and biomarkers such as urine, oral fluid, hair, and serum drug monitoring.

Clinical Outcomes

In the field of pain management, assessing adherence based on clinical outcomes is complex, as providers rely heavily on patient self-report, particularly regarding changes in pain intensity, which has been the gold standard since the 1996 American Pain Society's campaign to increase awareness for more effective pain care. This standard was subsequently adopted by the Department of Veterans Affairs and was a component of the Joint Commission on Accreditation of Healthcare Organization's "Standards Related to the Assessment and Treatment of Pain."[44] Recently, the use of pain intensity as an outcome measure has been challenged as being mis-leading, potentially contributing to inappropriate opioid use, and not fully capturing the multidimensional experience and impact of pain on the individual.[45] It may be more valid and meaningful to assess changes in mood and function as clinically relevant outcome measures using one of numerous validated measures of these domains.[23]

Patient Self-Report and Behavioral Measures

Multiple adherence assessment strategies have been employed, including patient self-report and tracking of behaviors or activities. For example, one approach is to simply ask the patients if they are using their medication and how they are using it, or if patients are following a home exercise program. Asking patients to keep a diary of their medication use or the frequency of performing a relaxation exercises can be effective in monitoring adherence. However, self-report measures tend to be inaccurate and subject to bias due to social desirability effects, as some patients strive to please their HCP or appear as "good" patients. Behavioral measures of adherence may include random pill counts, totaling the number of missed appointments for office visits, physical therapy, consultations and attendance for psychotherapy, or having the patient demonstrate a previously instructed therapy, exercise regimen, or use of a specific coping skill.

Biomarkers

The use of drug monitoring for specific patients can be a core component of a comprehensive opioid risk assessment and abuse mitigation program. There may be some utility in expanding drug monitoring as an adherence measure of other agents, such as antidepressants and anticonvulsants. This could provide the clinician with the opportunity to begin an open dialogue with the patient regarding his or her concerns about using these agents, such as issues of being stigmatized by others as a psychiatric patient if prescribed an antidepressant.

Unfortunately, there are no extant measurement instruments for adherence. In a meta-analysis by Hall et al.,[46] the authors reviewed measures of adherence to nonpharmacologic self-management treatments for chronic musculoskeletal pain. They found that measures of adherence can be grouped into home diaries, multi-item questionnaires, and single-item questionnaires and that all measures varied in the information assessed and scoring methodology and none met the rigors of appropriate psychometric test development. The authors concluded that while it is increasingly important to assess adherence, particularly to self-management interventions, there is a dearth of high-quality research in this area. Further research is needed in the area of measuring adherence to the wide range of interventions prescribed to patients with chronic pain.

INTERVENTIONS TO IMPROVE ADHERENCE IN PATIENTS WITH CHRONIC PAIN

CBT

Since CBT was introduced in the 1950s, primarily as a treatment for depression and anxiety disorders, it has expanded and been modified to include a number of treatments such as cognitive therapy, Acceptance and Commitment Therapy, rational-emotive behavior, dialectical behavior therapy, and mindfulness-based cognitive therapy and has been applied to a range of conditions such as posttraumatic stress disorders, bipolar disorders, eating disorders, personality disorders, insomnia, stress related to medical conditions, and pain management.[47] CBT can not only lead to improvement in primary pain management outcomes (mood, function) but also mitigate the risks for treatment nonadherence (pain, mood, sleep, substance misuse).

CBT for Chronic Pain

Patients with chronic pain often present with significant co-occurring depression and anxiety. Some patients with chronic pain engage in maladaptive behaviors (e.g., kinesiophobia, or fear of movement that will exacerbate pain; avoidance behaviors) and dysfunctional thinking patterns (e.g., catastrophizing). A number of psychological and behavioral therapies have demonstrated efficacy in improving chronic pain. These include acceptance/commitment therapy, which was discussed in chapter 2; mindfulness-based stress reduction programs; motivational interviewing; goal setting to enhance physical activation; opioid agreements; progressive muscle relaxation training, and CBT. CBT can include a number of these different strategies, with a process of identifying the maladaptive behaviors and/or dysfunctional thought patterns that may degrade the patient's ability to adjust to and cope with chronic pain.

CBT typically includes specific skill acquisition such as progressive muscle relaxation training, mindfulness-based stress reduction, and cognitive restructuring, followed by skill consolidation, rehearsal, and relapse training.[48] The process of cognitive restructuring consists of identifying and modifying negative thought patterns and substituting more rational cognitions to help the patient refrain and reconceptualize his or her own personal view of pain and encouraging the patient to be more proactive, rather than passive, and promoting a sense of competence and self-efficacy.

Cognitive therapy has been found to be cost-effective and clinically efficacious for a variety of chronic pain disorders including arthritis,[49] chronic low back pain,[50,51] lupus,[52] fibromyalgia,[53] and sickle cell disease.[54] A Cochrane Review by Bernardy et al.[55] evaluated the effectiveness of CBT for fibromyalgia, an often refractory condition. The authors evaluated 23 studies that met inclusion criteria with a total of 2,231 patients. Results indicated that CBT was superior to groups receiving a control condition in terms of reducing negative mood, decreasing disability, and pain reduction, both at treatment completion and six-months posttreatment completion.

CBT and Mood Disorders

Epidemiologic studies show that that depression and anxiety disorders are three to four times higher in chronic pain populations than base rates in the general population.[56] There is also robust evidence that depression strongly influences treatment adherence in a number of major medical disorders, including COPD,[57] hypertension,[58] HIV,[59] diabetes,[60] and coronary heart disease.[61] One theoretical model for explaining linkages between pain, depression, and nonadherence proposes that pain and pain-related disability lead to a state of depression, which in turn reduces adherence to therapeutic interventions, thus contributing to a cycle of continued pain and suffering (see Figure 6.2).

CBT is highly efficacious in treating depression. For example, a 2008 meta-analysis of randomized controlled trials (RBTs) of psychological interventions for major depressive disorders in primary care populations revealed that psychological interventions were more effective in improving depression compared to treatment as usual, when assessed at both short- and long-term time points. Psychological interventions were comparable to the effects of antidepressants.[62] In a large cohort study, 469 subjects meeting criteria for major depression who were refractory to antidepressant therapy were randomized into a treatment group that added a structured CBT program to the pharmacotherapy regimen or a treatment as usual group that received only continued antidepressant therapy (TAU). Patients were followed for 40 months on average from the completion of the trial. Results indicated that the group that received adjunctive CBT had statistically significantly improved depression scores that were sustained

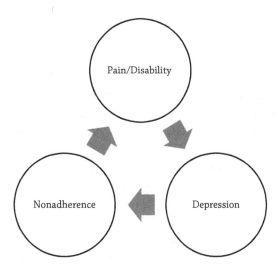

Figure 6.2. Pain-depression-nonadherence-pain cycle.

long-term as compared to the TAU group and that a cost analysis revealed substantial cost-effectiveness for adding the CBT to TAU.[63]

Patients who undergo CBT and other psychological therapies, such as Acceptance and Commitment Therapy and mindfulness-based stress reduction, can break the pain–depression–nonadherence cycle by targeting mood, pain coping skills, and physical activation, consequently improving adherence to other therapeutic interventions for chronic pain. The addition of an appropriately selected antidepressant can also enhance this therapeutic process.

CBT and Sleep Disorders

As noted earlier in this chapter, sleep disturbance is prevalent in patients with pain.[26,27] The association between persistent pain and sleep disturbance is bidirectional in nature[28,29] such that pain may lead to poor sleep quality and decreased total sleep time, therefore exacerbating pain and further impairing mood and contributing to decreased function and increased disability.[30,31] CBT has been employed to treat primary insomnia (CBT for insomnia [CBT-I]) and may confer distinct benefits to medications, including minimal adverse effects and targeting underlying mechanisms that can maintain chronic insomnia. A 2011 meta-analytic review of 14 randomized controlled trials (RCTs) that compared CBT-I to various control groups revealed that CBT-I had a medium to large effect size in improving in insomnia, and these effects were durable after the completion of treatment.[63] A subsequent systematic review by Mitchell et al.[64] identified five RCT studies that met criteria for inclusion that compared CBT-I to prescription and over-the-counter medications for sleep. The authors concluded that the data indicated that CBT-I was more effective than benzodiazepine and nonbenzodiazepine drugs in improving sleep and the effects may be more sustainable. This finding is particularly important in pain patients prescribed opioid analgesics as the risk for opioid-related fatalities significantly increases with the addition of a benzodiazepine.

A CBT-I treatment program typically includes six components: *psychoeducation* regarding sleep architecture and insomnia; *stimulus control* techniques to promote a strong association between the bed and rapid-onset sleep (e.g., removing the TV from the bedroom, restricting the use of bed for only sleep and sex, maintaining a regular wake/sleep cycle); *sleep restriction* (limiting the time spent in bed to only actual time asleep); *sleep hygiene* (targeting behaviors and environmental conditions that can promote or interfere with sleep such as timing of exercise, certain foods, bright lights, reading or watching material that is emotionally charged); *relaxation therapy* (reducing physical and mental tension via mediation, guided imagery, etc.); and *cognitive therapy* (addressing how beliefs and attitudes toward sleep can affect sleep-identify and replace maladaptive thoughts with rationale, adaptive ones).

Several studies have demonstrated the effectiveness of CBT-I in improving sleep in patients with pain.[65] There also has been interest in combining CBT-I and CBT for pain (CBT-P) into a hybrid program. Tang et al.[66] tested the feasibility and efficacy of a hybrid CBT-I and CBT-P program (CBT-I/P) in a cohort of 20 patients with chronic pain. The CBT-I/P resulted in improved sleep posttreatment and significantly greater reductions in depression, fatigue, and pain-related interference than a control group at both one- and six-month follow-ups. There was no change in pain intensity.

Cheatle et al. provide a comprehensive review of pain and sleep disturbance for the interested reader.[67]

CBT and Substance Abuse

Individuals who suffer from both pain and substance abuse tend to have higher degrees of depression, sleep disturbance, and anxiety that can dramatically reduce adherence to treatment for both disorders. There has also been significant concern regarding the burgeoning rate of prescription opioid misuse/abuse and opioid-related fatalities. The topics of effective risk assessment, monitoring, and mitigation strategies are beyond the scope of this chapter and have been discussed in detail in the literature. CBT, however, can be a useful tool in mitigating the risk of misuse and abuse in high-risk patients and in improving outcomes in patients with pain who have developed a substance use disorder (SUD). For example, in a recent study by Morasco et al.[68] patients with Hepatitis C virus, who had both chronic pain and SUD, were provided an eight-session integrated group CBT-P and SUD. The subjects completed a variety of standardized measures of pain, function, depression, and alcohol and substance use at baseline and posttreatment and also at three-month follow-up. Results from this pilot study revealed that there was improvement in pain interference, reduction in cravings for alcohol and other substances, and a decrease in past-month alcohol and substance use.

The process of CBT in addiction (and most likely pain) not only involves changing thoughts and behaviors but also altering brain function. There are evolving theories on the underlying neurobiological mechanisms of cognitive interventions in addiction. In a recent article by Zilverstand et al.,[69] the authors examined the literature on neuroimaging studies on cognitive interventions in addiction. They reviewed imaging studies involving CBT, cognitive inhibition of craving, motivational interventions, emotional regulation, mindfulness, and neurofeedback training in patients with addiction. Across all intervention modalities, there were common findings that included normalization of aberrant activity in the brain's reward circuitry and the recruitment and strengthening of the brain's inhibitory control network. Research along this line supports the efficacy of cognitive interventions for addiction and offers an opportunity for further investigation into the neurobiological mechanisms involved in the interaction of pain and addiction. This may provide new insights into this complex and treatment refractory patient population.

In summary, there is persuasive evidence that CBT is effective and efficacious in improving pain, sleep, mood, and substance misuse. Improvement in these conditions would facilitate adherence to other pain management interventions and support sustaining long-term improvements.

GOAL-SETTING AND BEHAVIOR CHANGE

Realistic goal setting can be a very powerful motivator in changing behaviors and maintaining the new behavior over time. One study by Tan et al.[70] demonstrated that individuals in a pain rehabilitation program that had specific return-to-work goals during their pain treatment program tended to have the highest probability of returning to gainful employment. In a study by Coppack et al.,[71] patients attending a residential rehabilitation program were randomized into an experimental exercise and goal-setting group, a therapist-led goal setting group, or a nontherapist-led exercise group. The experimental group had higher scores in self-efficacy as compared to the two other groups. Adherence to treatment was higher in the experimental group as compared to the nontherapist-led group but not the therapist-led exercise group. This study provided partial support of the benefit of goal setting and the effect of goal setting in improving patient self-efficacy, which also can be important in enhancing adherence.

Goals set by patients should be specific, quantifiable, realistic, and achievable, thus engendering a sense of self-efficacy and competence, and must be tied to meaningful rewards. Goal setting should be a dynamic not a static process, as the patient evolves through a treatment program.

BEHAVIORAL CONTRACTING

Another strategy that has been employed to improve adherence to a treatment regimen is developing a behavioral contract. This relies on having a strong HCP–patient relationship based on collaboration and open communication and involving the patient in the decision-making process. Contracting involves identifying well-defined behaviors that can lead to enhanced health and quality of life, such as nutritional changes, weight loss, exercise, and use of stress reduction techniques and through which fulfilling the contract results in tangible rewards, both intrinsic and extrinsic. Behavioral contracting has been used to improve adherence in a number of medical conditions, including hypertension, diabetes mellitus, and alcohol and drug treatment, among others.

A 2007 Cochrane review examined the effectiveness of contracts between patients and HCP in improving health outcomes, including adherence. The authors concluded that there was insufficient evidence that contracts improved adherence long term.[72] Contracting, however, provides an opportunity for the HCP to have an open discussion with the patient about what he or she perceives are important health behaviors to modify, which may be very divergent from ones identified by the HCP.

In pain medicine, opioid contracts are frequently used and are recommended as part of the standard of care when prescribing opioids for chronic noncancer pain. In this situation, using a contract allows the patient and HCP to define specific goals for opioid therapy such as increased activity, return to work or volunteering, or improved sleep or mood. Continued prescribing of opioids is contingent on reaching or movement toward specific goals. The contract also typically includes reasons for discontinuing opioids, agreeing to use one pharmacy, and not obtaining early refills, among other contingencies such as keeping appointments, bringing medications for pill counts, random urine screening, and so on. Although empirical data have not demonstrated increased adherence to a specified pharmacotherapy regimen or other components of a comprehensive pain treatment plan, the concrete communication channel opened up by, and documented through, this approach may enhance overall adherence.

SOCIAL SUPPORT

Social support has been postulated as a potentially important factor in improving adherence to treatment in a number of medical conditions. In a cross-sectional survey of medication adherence and associated factors for rural patients with hypertension, social support was a significant variable accounting for improved adherence to taking antihypertensive medications.[72] In a cohort of men receiving HIV treatment, receipt of recent social support was an important factor in predicting higher treatment self-efficacy, which in turn predicted medication and visit adherence.[73] Dunbar and Katz[74] performed a retrospective review of a group of patients with chronic pain and a history of SUD who were prescribed opioids. Patients who attended Alcoholics Anonymous (AA) regularly and had had an active support system had a lower rate of relapse than patients who had a poor support system. Many commercial weight loss programs rely heavily on social and peer support to enhance adherence to a weight loss program. Support obtained by attending AA, Narcotics Anonymous, and Overeaters Anonymous reinforces adherence to healthy lifestyles (abstinence, better nutrition), and social and peer support is a key component of group psychotherapy therapy to reinforce the adoption of new behaviors and attitudes.

Patients should be encouraged to bolster their social support while adopting and maintaining new behaviors or therapies to increase adherence through peer group membership, soliciting support from family and friends. Internet-based chat rooms or blogs may offer another source of support.

BARRIERS TO RECEIVING PSYCHOLOGICAL CARE

While psychological therapies may be effective in improving pain, mood, and function and address the risk factors for nonadherence, there are a number of barriers to receiving these needed services. Ehde et al.[75] out-lined some of these barriers, which included

- Financial (lack of insurance coverage for mental healthcare)
- Environmental (lack of transportation or lack of providers in the geographic region)
- Patient attitude-related (stigma associated with receiving psychological care)
- Healthcare systems barriers (no existing referral system to psychologists)

There are no easy answers to these barriers, and several researchers have suggested the potential to use nonpsychologists who otherwise routinely interact with patients to deliver CBT to their patients with pain. Examples might be dental hygienists for TMJ pain, physical and occupational therapists, certified nurse assistants, among others. While this may be potentially effective with some minimal training for less complex cases, a well-trained mental health provider is required for patients who have more complicated co-occurring mood and anxiety disorders. Improving reimbursement for psychological services and developing novel and high-quality delivery systems would help in addressing some of these barriers.

TELEHEALTH INTERVENTIONS

While the efficacy of CBT and other psychological interventions in improving mood, reducing risks, and promoting adherence is well established, access to these interventions is often limited due to the previously outlined barriers and availability of trained clinicians. There has been a movement to support improving access to these therapeutic interventions via e-health (delivering healthcare services via the Internet) and m-health (use of mobile phones) applications.

Computer-Assisted CBT for Pain and SUD

Internet-based CBT provides a structured course based on the same principles of face-to-face CBT but delivered through the Internet and can be either clinician guided or self-guided. Internet delivered CBT has been demonstrated as effective in improving certain aspects of pain conditions. Rini et al.[76] recently conducted a RCT comparing an automated Internet-based eight-week pain coping skills training program to a control group of patients with osteoarthritis pain. The experimental group had a high session completion adherence (91%) and overall reported significantly less pain as compared to the control group. Another study by Dear et al.[77] tested an enhanced clinician guided Internet-based CBT program for pain that included five sessions, homework assignments, weekly emails, or telephone contact with the clinical psychologist compared to a waitlist control group. Outcomes revealed that the treatment group had significantly greater improvements in anxiety, depression, average pain intensity, and disability as compared to the control group. The psychologists mean total time calling the subjects was 81.54 minutes.

Computerized CBT (cCBT) has also been demonstrated to be effective in improving treatment response and adherence in the very refractory population of patients with polysubstance abuse. Carroll et al.[78] evaluated the efficacy and utility of a cCBT training program (CBT4CBT) in 101 patients with cocaine use disorder maintained on methadone. Subjects were randomized into two groups, either standard methadone maintenance or methadone maintenance and weekly access to CBT4CBT. The CBT4CBT group had better outcomes than the methadone-only group with respect to weeks of abstinence from cocaine (36% vs. 17%) and urine specimens negative for all drugs. These improvements were generally maintained at six-month follow-up.

cCBT has the potential to broaden the availability of CBT to patients who may otherwise not be able to receive this type of treatment. Follow-up data suggest that cCBT is well accepted by patients.[79]

Telemedicine

Telemedicine has proved to be a very successful application to deliver health services to individuals in rural areas or who are unable to be seen in person due to either socioeconomic or physical barriers. Telemedicine provides face-to-face care through a direct, real-time video link to an individual patient or a group. Telemedicine has been employed in treating a range of medical and mental problems, even very complex conditions. For example, telemedicine was effective in treating posttraumatic stress disorder with prolonged exposure therapy to a group of veterans from the Afghanistan and Iraq conflicts.[80]

Smartphone Apps

A great deal of attention has been devoted to extending the use of smartphone apps from commercial/recreational use to healthcare delivery for mental health, including suicide prevention, addiction, and pain. A recent review of smartphone apps for mental health found 300 nonduplicate applications. The majority of apps claimed the purpose was symptom relief and general mental health education. Most apps provided no evidence of effectiveness of the app and no mention of security or privacy.[81] Another study explored the availability of smartphone apps for addiction recovery[82] and found 87 apps that contained information and tips on recovery from motivational tools to ways to promote social support and to monitor progress. App users expressed the opinion that the apps were useful in keeping them focused and inspired. The authors noted that few apps were formally evaluated by experts and more research was needed.

Larsen et al.[83] performed a systematic review of smartphone apps for suicide prevention. One hundred twenty-three apps were identified and reviewed. All of the reviewed apps had a least one suicide prevention strategy that was consistent with evidence-based or best practice guidelines, but some apps included potentially harmful content. The authors concluded that several apps may be useful but there was a need for further extensive research and development of more comprehensive and well-vetted apps for this patient population. Lallo et al.[84] discovered 279 pain management apps that met inclusion criteria for their review. None of the apps were comprehensive, and fewer than 10% of the apps included a HCP in the development or testing of the apps, and only one had been subjected to a scientific review.

While smartphone apps hold great promise to perhaps provide needed access to treatments for pain, mental health, and addiction, a great deal of research, development, and testing by a team of experts in technology, healthcare, law, and ethics are needed to ensure that disseminated apps are evidenced based and comprehensive and protect the rights and privacy of individuals. It is premature to relinquish the delivery of comprehensive treatment regimens, especially in complex and multifaceted conditions such as pain, to smartphone apps.

Currently smartphones may be best applied in improving adherence by providing prompts and reminders for certain behaviors such as keeping appointments, setting an alarm to take prescribed medications, track caloric intake, and physical activity.

Clinician Contact and e-Health

In this current healthcare climate of ever-expanding technologies and diminishing resources, it is tempting to overrely on e-health applications. In a recent review by Newman et al.[86] of technology-assisted self-help and minimal-contact therapies for mood and anxiety disorders, the authors concluded that while therapist-assisted treatments remain optimal in the treatment of more significant cases of depression, self-help cCBT interventions are efficacious only in the treatment of subthreshold mood disorders. In a review by the same authors on technology-assisted self-help therapies for drug and alcohol abuse, similar results were obtained. In treating patient with SUDs, self-administered and predominantly self-help cCBT interventions can be efficacious, but some therapist contact is critical for more sustained reductions in addictive behavior.[87]

CONCLUSIONS

In the current healthcare climate, HCPs are faced with multiple competing demands of increased productivity, navigating electronic medical record systems, fulfilling regulatory requirements (e.g., "meaningful use"), extensive documentation of care, following ever-expanding clinical guidelines, cost-containment, and ensuring patient satisfaction. Patient nonadherence to prescribed therapeutics and changes in health behaviors adds another layer of frustration to the busy HCP. While most HCPs are cognizant that a positive HCP–patient relationship is pivotal in improving both adherence to treatment recommendations and patient satisfaction, the copious and increasing responsibilities placed on HCPs in daily practice often leave little time to foster this relationship. Additional barriers to improving adherence include deficiencies in teaching adherence techniques during training, institutional/environmental obstacles (crowded and hectic clinics, mandated increase productivity), limited or no access to psychological services, and the socioeconomic barriers faced by patients.

Meaningful changes in HCP training, accessibility and affordability of needed services, and improved reimbursement for noninterventional HCPs and treatments are required if adherence to evidence-based, efficacious therapies for chronic pain and other major medical disorders is to improve. The ever-evolving and expanding use of e-health applications provide promise for addressing some of these issues but demand further evaluation and testing by content experts. The greatest tool in improving adherence, however, is the HCP–patient relationship and the attitude of the HCP toward the patient and his or her circumstances.

> The good physician treats the disease; the great physician treats the patient who has the disease.
>
> William Osler

REFERENCES

1. Tsang A, Von Korff M, Lee S, et al. Common chronic pain conditions in developed and developing countries: gender and age differences and comorbidity with depression-anxiety disorders. *J Pain.* 2008;9(10):883–891.
2. Johannes CB, Kim Le T, Zhou X, Johnston JA, Dworkin RH. The prevalence of chronic pain in United States adults: results of an Internet-based survey. *J Pain.* 2010;11(11):1230–1239.
3. Institute of Medicine. *Relieving Pain in America: A Blueprint for Transforming Prevention, Care, Education, and Research: A Call for Public Action.* Washington, DC: National Academies Press; 2011.
4. Peppin JF, Cheatle MD, Kirsh KL, McCarberg BH. The complexity model: a novel approach to improve chronic pain care. *Pain Med.* 2015;16(4):653–666.
5. Jamison RN. Nonspecific treatment effects in pain medicine. *ISAP Pain Clin Updates.* 2011;19(2):1–7.
6. Turk DC, Swanson K. Efficacy and cost-effectiveness treatment of chronic pain: an analysis and evidence-based synthesis. In: Schatman ME, Campbell A, eds. *Chronic Pain Management: Guidelines for Multidisciplinary Program Development.* New York: Informa Healthcare; 2007:15–38.
7. Oslund S, Robinson RC, Clark TC, et al. Long-term effectiveness of a comprehensive pain management program: strengthening the case for interdisciplinary care. *Proc (Bayl Univ Med Cent).* 2009;22(3):211–214.
8. Cheatle MD, Gallagher RM. Chronic pain and comorbid mood and substance use disorders: a biopsychosocial treatment approach. *Curr Psychiatry Rep.* 2006;8(5):371–376.
9. Cheatle, MD. Biopsychosocial approach to assessing and managing patients with chronic pain. *Med Clin North Am.* 2016;100(1):43–53.
10. Sabaté E, ed. *Adherence to Long-Term Therapies: Evidence for Action.* Geneva: World Health Organization; 2003.
11. Farin E, Gramm L, Schmidt E. The patient–physician relationship in patients with chronic low back pain as a predictor of outcomes after rehabilitation. *J Behav Med.* 2013;36(3):246–258.
12. Farin E, Nagl M. The patient–physician relationship in patients with breast cancer: influence on changes in quality of life after rehabilitation. *Qual Life Res.* 2013;22(2):283–294.
13. Timmerman L, Stronks DL, Groeneweg JG, Huygen FJ. Prevalence and determinants of medication non-adherence in chronic pain patients: a systematic review. *Acta Anaesthesiol Scand.* 2016;60(4):416–431.

14. Prochaska JO, DiClemente CC. Stages of change in the modification of problem behaviors. *Prog Behav Modif.* 1992;28:183–218.
15. Gentil L, Vasilliadis H, Preville M, Bosse C, Berbiche D. Association between depressive and anxiety disorders and adherence to antihypertensive medication in community-living elderly adults. *J Am Geriatr Soc.* 2012;60(12):2297–2301.
16. Albrecht JS, Park Y, Hur P, et al. Adherence to maintenance medications among older adults with chronic obstructive pulmonary disease: the role of depression. *Ann Am Thorac Soc.* 2016;13(9):1497–1504.
17. Gonzalez JS, Batchelder AW, Psaros C, Safren SA. Depression and HIV/AIDS treatment nonadherence: a review and meta-analysis. *J Acquir Immune Defic Syndr.* 2011;58(2):181–187.
18. Cabrera-Marroquín R, Contreras-Yáñez I, Alcocer-Castillejos N, Pascual-Ramos V. Major depressive episodes are associated with poor concordance with therapy in rheumatoid arthritis patients: the impact on disease outcomes. *Clin Exp Rheumatol.* 2014;32(6):904–913.
19. Kroenke K, Spitzer RL, Williams JB. The PHQ-9: validity of a brief depression severity measure. *J Gen Intern Med.* 2001;16(9):606–613.
20. Zung W. A self-rating depression scale. *Arch Gen Psychiatry.*1965;12:63–70.
21. Beck AT, Epstein N, Brown G, Steer RA. An inventory for measuring clinical anxiety: psychometric properties. *J Consult Clin Psychol.* 1988;56(6):893–7.
22. Bjelland L, Dahl AA, Haug TT, Neckelmann D. The validity of the Hospital Anxiety and Depression Scale. An updated literature review. *J Psychosom Res.* 2002;52(1):69–77.
23. Dworkin RH, Turk DC, Farrar JT, et al. Core outcome measures for chronic pain trials: IMMPACT recommendations. *Pain.* 2005;113(1–2):9–19.
24. Beck A, Ward C, Mendelson M, Mock J, Erbaugh J. An inventory for measuring depression. *Arch Gen Psychiatry.* 1961;4:561–571.
25. McNair D, Lorr M, Droppleman L. *Profile of Mood States.* San Diego, CA: Educational and Industrial Testing Service; 1971.
26. Tang NK, Wright KJ, Salkovskis PM. Prevalence and correlates of clinical insomnia co-occurring with chronic back pain. *J Sleep Res.* 2007;16(1):85–95.
27. McCracken LM, Williams JL, Tang NK. Psychological flexibility may reduce insomnia in persons with chronic pain: a preliminary retrospective study. *Pain Med.* 2011;12(6):904–912.
28. Sivertsen B, Lallukka T, Petrie KJ, Steingrímsdóttir ÓA, Stubhaug A, Nielsen CS. Sleep and pain sensitivity in adults. *Pain.* 2015;156(8): 1433–1439.
29. Moldofsky H, Lue FA, Eisen J, Keystone E, Gorczynski RM. The relationship of interleukin-1 and immune functions to sleep in humans. *Psychosom Med.* 1986;48(5):309–318.
30. Haythornthwaite JA, Hegel MT, Kerns RD. Development of a sleep diary for chronic pain patients. *J Pain Symptom Manage.* 1991;6(2):65–72.
31. Chiu YH, Silman AJ, Macfarlane GJ, et al. Poor sleep and depression are independently associated with a reduced pain threshold. Results of a population based study. *Pain.* 2005;115(3):316–321.
32. Wolff BB. Evaluation of hypnotics in outpatients with insomnia using a questionnaire and a self-rating technique. *Clin Pharmacol Ther.* 1974;15:130–140
33. Buysse DJ, Reynolds CF 3rd, Monk TH, Berman SR, Kupfer DJ. The Pittsburgh Sleep Quality Index: a new instrument for psychiatric practice and research. *Psychiatry Res.* 1989;28(2):193–213.

34. Moul DE, Hall M, Pilkonis PA, Buysse DJ. Self-report measures of insomnia in adults: rationales, choices, and needs. *Sleep Med Rev.* 2004;8(3):177–198.

35. Frier A, Barnett F, Devine S. The relationship between social determinants of health, and rehabilitation of neurological conditions: a systematic literature review. *Disabil Rehabil.* 2016 May 22:1–8.

36. Webster LR, Webster RM. Predicting aberrant behaviors in opioid-treated patients: preliminary validation of the Opioid Risk Tool. *Pain Med.* 2005;6:432–442.

37. Butler S, Budman S et al. Validation of a screener and opioid assessment measure for patients with chronic pain. *Pain.* 2004;112(1–2):65–75.

38. Belgrade M, Schamber C, Lindgren B. The DIRE score: predicting outcomes of opioid prescribing for chronic pain. *J Pain* 2006;7(9):671–681.

39. Skinner HA. The drug abuse screening test. *Addict Behav.* 1982;7(4):363–371.

40. Passik S, Kirsh KL, Whitcomb L, et al. A new tool to assess and document pain outcomes in chronic pain patients receiving opioid therapy. *Clin Ther.* 2004;26 (4):552–561.

41. Butler S, Budman SH, Fernandez KC, et al. Development and validation of the Current Opioid Misuse Measure. *Pain.* 2007;130 (1–2):144–156.

42. Brown RL, Rounds LA. Conjoint screening questionnaires for alcohol and other drug abuse: criterion validity in a primary care practice. *Wis Med J.* 1995;94(3):135–140

43. Chou R, Fanciullo GJ, Fine PG, Miaskowski C, Passik SD, Portenoy RK. Opioids for chronic noncancer pain: prediction and identification of aberrant drug-related behaviors: a review of the evidence for an American Pain Society and American Academy of Pain Medicine clinical practice guideline. *J Pain.* 2009;10(2): 131–146.

44. Phillips DM. JCAHO pain management standards are unveiled. *JAMA.* 2000;284:428–429.

45. Ballantyne JC, Sullivan MD. Intensity of chronic pain. *N Engl J Med.* 2016;374(14):1395.

46. Hall AM, Kamper SJ, Hernon M, et al. Measurement tools for adherence to non-pharmacologic self-management treatment for chronic musculoskeletal conditions: a systematic review. *Arch Phys Med Rehabil.* 2015;96(3):552–562.

47. Hollon SD, Beck AT. Cognitive and cognitive behavioral-therapies. In Lambert M, ed. *Bergin and Garfield's Handbook of Psychotherapy and Behavior Change,* 6th ed. Hoboken, NJ. John Wiley:393–542.

48. Turk DC, Flor H. Etiological theories and treatments for chronic back pain. II. Psychological models and interventions. *Pain.* 1984;19(3):209–233.

49. Keefe FJ, Caldwell DS. Cognitive behavioral control of arthritis pain. *Med Clin North Am.* 1997;81:277–290.

50. Linton SJ. A 5-year follow-up evaluation of the health and economic consequences of an early cognitive behavioral intervention for back pain: a randomized, controlled trial. *Spine.* 2006;31(8):853–858.

51. Lamb SE, Hansen Z, Lall R, Castelnuovo E, Withers EJ, Nichols V. Group cognitive behavioral treatment for low-back pain in primary care: a randomized controlled trial and cost-effectiveness analysis. *Lancet.* 2010;375:916–923.

52. Greco CM, Rudy TE, Manzi S. Effects of a stress-reduction program on psychological function, pain, and physical function of systemic lupus erythematosus patients: a randomized controlled trial. *Arthritis Rheum.* 2004; 51(4)625–634.

53. Thieme K, Flor H, Turk D. Psychological pain treatment in fibromyalgia syndrome: efficacy of operant behavioral and cognitive behavioral treatments. *Arthritis Res Ther.* 2006;8(4):R121.
54. Chen E, Cole SW, Kato PM. A review of empirically supported psychosocial interventions for pain and adherence outcomes in sickle cell disease. *J Pediatr Psychol.* 2004;29:1997–2009.
55. Bernardy K, Klose P, Busch AJ, Choy EH, Häuser W. Cognitive behavioural therapies for fibromyalgia. *Cochrane Database Syst Rev.* 2013;10(9):CD009796. doi:10.1002/14651858.CD009796.pub2.
56. Magni G, Marchetti M, Moreschi C, Merskey H, Luchini S. Chronic musculoskeletal pain and depressive symptoms in the National Health and Nutrition Examination, I: epidemiologic follow-up study. *Pain* 1993;53(2):163–168.
57. Albrecht JS, Park Y, Hur P, et al. Adherence to maintenance medications among older adults with chronic obstructive pulmonary disease: the role of depression. *Ann Am Thorac Soc.* 2016;13(9):1497–1504.
58. Perez-Cornago A, Sanchez-Villegas A, Bes-Rastrollo M, et al. Relationship between adherence to Dietary Approaches to Stop Hypertension (DASH) diet indices and incidence of depression during up to 8 years of follow-up. *Public Health Nutr.* 2016 Jun 23:1–10.
59. Starace F, Ammassari A, Trotta MP, et al. Depression is a risk factor for suboptimal adherence to highly active antiretroviral therapy. *J Acquir Immune Defic Syndr.* 2002;31:S136–S139.
60. Capoccia K, Odegard PS, Letassy N. Medication adherence with diabetes medication: a systematic review of the literature. *Diabetes Educ.* 2016;42(1):34–71.
61. Gehi A, Haas D, Pipkin S, Whooley MA. Depression and medication adherence in outpatients with coronary heart disease. *Arch Intern Med.* 2005;165(21):2508–2513.
62. Bortolotti B, Menchetti M, Bellini F, Montaguti MB, Berardi D. Psychological interventions for major depression in primary care: a meta-analytic review of randomized controlled trials. *Gen Hosp Psychiatry.* 2008;30(4):293–302.
63. Wiles NJ, Thomas L, Turner N, et al. Long-term effectiveness and cost-effectiveness of cognitive behavioural therapy as an adjunct to pharmacotherapy for treatment-resistant depression in primary care: follow-up of the CoBalT randomised controlled trial. *Lancet Psychiatry.* 2016;3(2):137–144.
64. Okajima I, Komada Y, Inoue Y. A meta-analysis on the treatment effectiveness of cognitive behavioral therapy for primary insomnia. *Sleep Biol Rhythms.* 2011;9:24–34.
65. Mitchell MD, Gehrman P, Perlis M, Umscheid CA. Comparative effectiveness of cognitive behavioral therapy for insomnia: a systematic review. *BMC Fam Pract.* 2012;13:40.
66. Jungquist CR, Tra Y, Smith MT, et al. The durability of cognitive behavioral therapy for insomnia in patients with chronic pain. *Sleep Discord.* 2012:679648.
67. Tang NK, Goodchild CE, Salkovskis PM. Hybrid cognitive-behavior therapy for individuals with insomnia and chronic pain: a pilot randomized controlled trial. *Behav Res Ther.* 2012;50(12):814–821.
68. Cheatle MD, Foster S, Pinkett A, Lesneski M, Qu D, Dhingra L. Assessing and managing sleep disturbance in patients with chronic pain. *Anesthesiol Clin.* 2016;34(2):379–393.
69. Morasco BJ, Greaves DW, Lovejoy TI, Turk DC, Dobscha SK, Hauser P. Development and preliminary evaluation of an integrated cognitive-behavior

treatment for chronic pain and substance use disorder in patients with the hepatitis C virus. *Pain Med.* 2016 Jun 2;pii: pnw076. [Epub ahead of print]

70. Zilverstand A, Parvaz MA, Moeller SJ, Goldstein RZ. Cognitive interventions for addiction medicine: understanding the underlying neurobiological mechanisms. *Prog Brain Res.* 2016;224:285–304.

71. Tan V, Cheatle MD, Mackin S, Moberg PJ, Esterhai JL Jr. Goal setting as a predictor of return to work in a population of chronic musculoskeletal pain patients. *Int J Neurosci.* 1997;92(3–4):161–170.

72. Coppack RJ, Kristensen J, Karageorghis CI. Use of a goal setting intervention to increase adherence to low back pain rehabilitation: a randomized controlled trial. *Clin Rehabil.* 2012;26(11):1032–1042.

73. Bosch-Capblanch X, Abba K, Prictor M, Garner P. Contracts between patients and healthcare practitioners for improving patients' adherence to treatment, prevention and health promotion activities. *Cochrane Database Syst Rev.* 2007;18(2):CD004808.

74. Ganguli A, Clewell J, Shillington AC. The impact of patient support programs on adherence, clinical, humanistic, and economic patient outcomes: a targeted systematic review. *Patient Prefer Adherence.* 2016;10:711–725.

75. Turan B, Fazeli PL, Raper JL, Mugavero MJ, Johnson MO. Social support and moment-to-moment changes in treatment self-efficacy in men living with HIV: Psychosocial moderators and clinical outcomes. *Health Psychol.* 2016 Apr 18. [Epub ahead of print]

76. Dunbar SA, Katz NP. Chronic opioid therapy for nonmalignant pain in patients with a history of substance abuse: report of 20 cases. *J Pain Symptom Manage.* 1996;11(3):163–171.

77. Ehde DM, Dillworth TM, Turner JA. Cognitive-behavioral therapy for individuals with chronic pain: efficacy, innovations, and directions for research. *Am Psychol.* 2014;69(2):153–166.

78. Rini C, Porter LS, Somers TJ, et al. Automated Internet-based pain coping skills training to manage osteoarthritis pain: a randomized controlled trial. *Pain.* 2015;156(5):837–848.

79. Dear BF, Titov N, Perry KN, et al. The Pain Course: a randomized controlled trial of a clinician-guided Internet-delivered cognitive behavior therapy program for managing chronic pain and emotional well-being. *Pain.* 2013;154(6):942–950.

80. Carroll KM, Kiluk BD, Nich C, et al. Computer-assisted delivery of cognitive-behavioral therapy: efficacy and durability of CBT4CBT among cocaine-dependent individuals maintained on methadone. *Am J Psychiatry.* 2014;171(4):436–444.

81. National Institute for Health and Clinical Excellence. Computerized cognitive behavior therapy for depression and anxiety: Review of technology appraisal 51 (Technology Appraisal 97); 2006. Available at http://www.nice.org.uk/nicemedia/pdf/TA097guidance.pdf. Accessed August 17, 2011.

82. Tuerk PW, Yoder M, Ruggiero K, Gros DF, Acierno R. A pilot study of prolonged exposure therapy for posttraumatic stress disorder delivered via telehealth technology. *J Traumatic Stress.* 2010;23:116–123.

83. Radovic A, Vona PL, Santostefano AM, Ciaravino S, Miller E, Stein BD. Smartphone applications for mental health. *Cyberpsychol Behav Soc Netw.* 2016;19(7):465–470.

84. Savic M, Best D, Rodda S, Lubman DI. Exploring the focus and experiences of smartphone applications for addiction recovery. *J Addict Dis.* 2013;32(3):310–319.

85. Larsen ME, Nicholas J, Christensen H. A Systematic assessment of smartphone tools for suicide prevention. *PLoS One.* 2016;11(4):e0152285.

86. Lalloo C, Jibb LA, Rivera J, Agarwal A, Stinson JN. "There's a pain app for that": review of patient-targeted smartphone applications for pain management. *Clin J Pain.* 2015;31(6):557–563.

87. Newman MG, Szkodny LE, Llera SJ, Przeworski A. A review of technology-assisted self-help and minimal contact therapies for anxiety and depression: is human contact necessary for therapeutic efficacy? *Clin Psychol Rev.* 2011;31(1):89–103.

88. Newman MG, Szkodny LE, Llera SJ, Przeworski A. A review of technology-assisted self-help and minimal contact therapies for drug and alcohol abuse and smoking addiction: is human contact necessary for therapeutic efficacy? *Clin Psychol Rev.* 2011;31(1):178–186.

CHAPTER 7

⚬∿⚬

Adherence in Pain Medicine

Ethical Considerations

MICHAEL E. SCHATMAN AND OSCAR J. BENITEZ

INTRODUCTION

Adherence has been defined by the World Health Organization as "the extent to which a person's behavior—taking medication, following a diet, and/or executing lifestyle changes, corresponds with agreed recommendations from a health care provider."[1(p17)] Due to increased regulatory scrutiny and clinician wariness regarding sanctions, however, *adherence* in pain medicine specifically has devolved over the past decade simply into compliance with opioid prescriptions and policies.[2,3] Although few would argue that adherence to opioid prescription is not a crucial concern, focusing exclusively on this issue results in a failure to recognize that pain medicine is more than prescribing and monitoring opioid therapy and that adherence is a more global phenomenon that involves the necessity of patients with pain and their clinicians establishing a trusting partnership following if they are to make meaningful, health-improving strides in regard to persistent pain and its sequelae.

This chapter examines adherence from the perspective of principle-based ethics as described by Beauchamp and Childress,[4] which maintains that clinical appropriateness can be determined through the four tenets of autonomy, nonmaleficence, beneficence, and justice. Beauchamp and

Childress have maintained that these four principles can explain and justify, alone or in combination, all the substantive and universal claims of medical ethics, and probably of ethics more generally. No principle is absolutely binding; it may be superseded in a situation by an equal or more applicable principle.[5]

PATIENT AUTONOMY

The literature on ethical issues associated with medical adherence has focused heavily on respect for patient autonomy—that is, a patient's right to determine what treatment he or she receives,[6–8] with this same focus consistently evident in the literature on adherence in pain medicine.[9,10] Many believe that respect for patient autonomy is the cornerstone not only of principle-based ethics but also that of the ethical practice of medicine, generally.[11–13] This strong regard for the primacy of autonomy is based, in part, on the belief that it is a necessary component of nonmaleficence, beneficence, and justice.[14] In order to understand the ethical implications of respect for patient autonomy in pain medicine, the concept needs to be examined more closely as it relates to the current realities of the larger systems of care in which the pain management is subsumed.

As conceptualized by the ancient Greeks, medical decision-making should be a process that occurs solely within the sacred covenant of the patient–clinician dyad.[15] Unfortunately, so-call third-party stakeholders, such as the health insurance industry, have become inextricable decision-makers in pain medicine in the United States, influencing heavily (and some would aver negatively) the quality of care that patients with pain receive.[16]. The ethical implications of this occurrence is that when the "profession" of pain medicine devolves to the "business" of pain medicine autonomy—expressed as patient-centric care with the best interests of the patient as the imperative—is stripped away.[17] On the other hand, Roter[18] has posited that we are evidencing a progressive shift in power in the patient–clinician relationship, with an emphasis on shared decision-making becoming progressively more strongly embraced. For many years, shared decision-making has been considered an important strategy for reducing the informational and power asymmetry that has traditionally existed between clinicians and patients.[19] The shift to shared decision-making as a realization of autonomy in medical practice over the past few decades stands in contrast to the long-held traditional paternalistic model—which disempowered the patient.[20]

Medical Decision-Making

Few would argue that competent patients have the "right" to determine whether or not to have pain treated and to agree or not with recommendations made by their clinicians. However, the question of how much say a patient without known risk factors should have in treatment decisions, especially regarding controlled substances, and opioids in particular, needs to be considered. American pain medicine has recently witnessed a dramatic shift from a period of liberal opioid prescribing to wariness and pull-back.[21,22] Physician practices and health systems have adopted policies discouraging chronic opioid therapy for noncancer pain conditions, in part based on recently revised opioid prescribing guidelines.[23] We posit that well-selected and adherent patients should be provided the option of opioid therapy if other options are contraindicated, pose greater risk than opioids, are likely to be or have been ineffective, or are unavailable (e.g., due to insurance company refusal to pay for safer, more evidence-based treatments).[16] For the clinician willing to consider chronic opioid therapy, however, a significant factor in adherence is the provision of genuine informed consent regarding the iatrogenic complications of such treatment. Although commonly utilized in pain medicine, opioid agreements are typically unilateral—replete with "thou shalt" and "thou shalt not" statements regarding expectations of the patient. Accordingly, they have been criticized as "alienating" and thereby potentially deleterious to the clinician-patient relationship.[24] What most agreements lack, unfortunately, is information regarding iatrogeneses such as opioid-induced endocrinopathy, which has become an empirically demonstrated complication of chronic opioid use.[25] In the absence of demonstrated aberrant medication use, should a patient have a degree of self-determination regarding whether the analgesia that may be obtained from ongoing opioid therapy is or is not more important than is the likelihood of his or her encountering adverse effects?. The ethical principle of autonomy is contingent upon the doctrine of informed consent,[26] and physicians who treat chronic pain should have respect for the phenomenological experiences and informed choices of their patients.

The Issue of Excessive Autonomy

Aside from opioids, it appears that patients with chronic pain are perhaps given *excessive* autonomy when demonstrating poor treatment adherence. For example, tobacco smokers routinely undergo elective spinal surgery, despite the empirical literature indicating that smokers respond more poorly to surgery than do nonsmokers.[27-29] Given the recent review[30] indicating that a substantial number of patients undergoing spinal surgery experience *increased* pain and disability at one- and two-year follow-ups, should surgeons perform these surgeries on patients who do not demonstrate adherence by discontinuing their tobacco use? Curiously, as surgeons understand the deleterious impact of smoking on surgical outcomes, perhaps it is *their* adherence that should be questioned. Certainly, the overperformance of spine surgeries may be in part driven by the profit motive,[31] which is an example of a pitfall of "pay for procedures" trumping "pay for performance" in the American healthcare system. Similarly, are patients who are "prescribed" physical therapy required to demonstrate adherence? Physical therapy, in the form of specifically guided and instructed but largely self-directed physical activities (stretching, strengthening, movement, and cardiovascular fitness, etc.) for patients with chronic pain, should not be considered "treatment" but rather "self-management training." Adherence not only requires that patients complete assigned exercise programs on days on which they do not attend a formal physical therapy session but recognizes the imperative of adopting exercise into their daily lives on an ongoing basis.[32-34] At face value, guidelines for treatment that stipulate discharge from a pain management program for failure to follow through with assigned exercise programs might seem sound, this type of nonadherence and its consequences have ethical implications superimposed on clinical outcomes alone. Nonadherence in patients with chronic pain obviously and inevitably results in "treatment failure," further demoralizing a patient population that is already psychologically vulnerable.[35] The ethical clinician has a duty to balance "autonomy" (nonadherence) with nonmaleficence (doing no harm), explicitly reconciling these two principles on behalf of the best interests of the patient. Again, in support of autonomy, this is best carried out through direct and open communication with the patient in a nonconfrontational manner. In fact, this approach has been shown to be one of the more powerful means to instill and strengthen trust, one of the most powerful "levers" to enhance adherence.[36]

Balancing Patient Autonomy and Paternalism

There is clear tension between respect for patient autonomy and the conflicting position of traditional paternalism in medicine,[37] and this discordance has significant implications for patient adherence in pain medicine.

The paternalistic assumption is that the clinician knows best.[38] McKinstry[39] has noted that there are actually two types of paternalism. The most severe is the "autocratic" physician, who has little concern for the opinions of the patient. The second type is the paternalistic physician who will listen to the patient but sees him- or herself as "superior" to the patient and is accordingly comfortable in overriding the patient's wishes. The American healthcare system, including pain medicine, has been in a state of crisis for a number of years,[17,40–42] with pain medicine's status as a discipline not yet fully incorporated into the mainstream.[43] This is a potential cause of the dramatic shortage of pain management specialists in the United States.[44] When society in general, and medical practitioners in particular, marginalize a population such as those living with chronic pain, it results in what Cohen and colleagues have labeled the "extinction of empathy."[45] In pain medicine, empathy is critical, as it allows patients to more healthfully adapt to the inevitable frustrations that are part and parcel of living this "invisible" condition.[46]

The paternalistic model fails to respect the phenomenological experience of the patient. In pain medicine, no less than any other cohort of patients, lumping all people with chronic pain together as a homogeneous population results in missing each individual's unique biopsychosocial experience of pain. Doing so is dehumanizing and has been postulated to increase patient suffering.[47] An increasingly common situation that occurs within the current climate of questioning the potential benefits of opioids as a legitimate and potentially useful therapeutic tool in the management of certain patients with chronic pain conditions is clinician–patient disagreement regarding the ultimate goal of pain medicine.[48] If a patient is primarily interested in analgesia and his or her physician is primarily invested in increasing the patient's functional capacity, whose objective should win out? Although the principle of respect for patient autonomy would suggest that patients without a substance use disorder should have a voice (i.e., exercise autonomy) in whether he or she should be prescribed opioid analgesia, a reversion to a more paternalistic stance with regard to chronic opioid therapy contravenes such a point of view. When patients with chronic pain request opioid analgesics and focus on analgesia rather than functionality, they are likely be seen as "nonadherent"—and often accused of being addicted to pain medications. Clearly, this type of paternalism, in the absence of more objective patient-specific data to inform care planning, can have negative emotional consequences as well as physical consequences for patients suffering from chronic pain.

NONMALEFICENCE

Nonmaleficence refers to the duty of the healthcare practitioner to avoid causing harm to a patient, whether it is intentional or inadvertent. Based on the concept of *primum non nocere*,[49] few would argue that clinicians are not obligated to do their best to prevent harm. There are undoubtedly many instances in which demanding adherence prevents patients with chronic pain from being harmed. Given the more than 18,000 unintentional prescription opioid-related deaths that occurred in the United States in 2014,[50] requiring patient adherence in regard to medication and substance use is an imperative. Nonadherence to accepted risk mitigation practices by prescribing clinicians is an equally paramount issue that must be confronted in order to reduce serious harms associated with prescription opioids.[51-55]

Psychological Assessment of the Risk of Substance Misuse and Abuse

The majority of the universal precautions elucidated by Gourlay and colleagues[52] more than a decade ago have evidence bases for increasing the safety of opioid prescribing, which makes clinicians' nonadherence to them particularly maleficent. For example, the authors recommend that patients are provided with a psychological assessment, including risk of addictive disorders. This is indeed important, as empirical data indicate that psychological conditions such as depression[56] and anxiety[57] are risk factors for opioid aberrancy. Although a pain psychology evaluation would be ideal to identify psychological risk factors prior to prescribing opioids, the shortage of qualified pain psychologists—particularly in underserved areas—leave physicians (and their patients in need of safe and effective pain care) on their own.[58] However, a number of screening tools for depression and anxiety exist that have been validated in the chronic pain population[59-62] that can be quickly and easily administered, scored, and interpreted by physicians and their office staffs in order to identify these psychological factors. How frequently are such measures utilized as screening tools in medical practices prior to prescribing opioids? Although we were unable to identify reliable data indicating their prevalence of utilization, our clinical experience tells us that such screening is rare. Similarly, well-validated measures developed specifically to stratify patients' risks for aberrant use of opioids exist and are available at no cost online, and most are extremely user-friendly.[63] Unfortunately, these types of measures are underutilized in clinical practice—thereby leaving prescribers less informed and patients considered for opioid therapy at potentially greater risk than need be. This is an example of adherence being the proverbial knife that cuts both ways, necessarily involving clinician and patient.

Monitoring the Four A's of Pain Medicine

Another example of universal precautions, likely to go unheeded and potentially resulting in harm to patients, is monitoring of the Four A's" (analgesia, activity, adverse effects, and aberrant behavior) of pain medicine.[64] One would logically conclude that a clinician prescribing a Schedule II medication would see a patient on a monthly basis and monitor analgesia, activity levels, and adverse effects closely. Does this routinely happen in clinical practice? A search of the literature fails to yield evidence that this is the case. There is clearly considerable variance in the extent to which clinicians exercise due diligence in their opioid prescribing practices, and many of our patients complain that their well-being becomes an "afterthought" once they begin chronic opioid therapy. For example, despite data indicating that as many as 81% of patients taking opioids for chronic pain experience opioid-induced constipation,[65] many physicians lack awareness of this side effect, and many who are aware fail to ask their patients whether they are experiencing this distressing and highly predictable and preventable adverse effect.[66] This is particularly problematic in regard to the harm to patients whose constipation secondary to opioids experience more than just physical discomfort. Coyne and colleagues[67] found that among patients with opioid-induced constipation, 9% reported missing work due to their symptoms and 38% experienced activity impairment. Results of another study indicate that among patients with chronic pain on opioids, constipation was predictive of more hospitalizations and emergency department visits.[68] Finally, patients with opioid-induced constipation are more likely to reduce their dosage of pain medication in order to reduce their bowel dysfunction, potentially resulting in oligoanalgesia, or less than plausibly optimal pain control.[69]

It is critical for clinicians to adhere to monitoring another of the Four A's, aberrant behavior. The harms that this lack of adherence causes both individuals and society as a whole are certainly obvious. Urine drug testing (UDT) is far from a "cure" for aberrant drug taking behaviors. However, in reviewing the literature, its efficacy for detecting inappropriate use of opioids, as well as other substances, is limited (see chapter 4). Deyo and colleagues[70] recently noted that screening for high-risk patients, treatment agreements, and UDT have not reduced rates of opioid prescribing, misuse, or overdose. However, what this review does not address is how much more severe the opioid crisis would potentially have become without tools such as UDT. Although certainly not a panacea, myriad reviews[71-87] have supported the utility of UDT when applied appropriately as an aspect of a *comprehensive* risk mitigation approach and as an important tool in the prevention of aberrant drug use. Unfortunately, many clinicians are not adherent with guidelines recommending UDT for patients receiving chronic opioid therapy. For example, in a 2013 study of primary care opioid prescribing in a Veterans Affairs Medical Center, only half of patients on chronic opioid therapy underwent urine drug monitoring.[88] In a civilian teaching hospital, a recent study of guideline concordance found that almost half of patients with chronic noncancer pain on long-term opioid therapy who were treated by resident physicians, and approximately a third of patients who were treated by attending physicians, failed to receive urine drug screening.[89] Most discouraging are results of a study of patients with chronic pain determined to be at high risk for problematic drug use in which only 8% underwent UDT.[90] However, results of a study by Morasco and colleagues[91] of chronic noncancer pain patients being treated at a Veterans Affairs health system clinic were somewhat more encouraging, indicating that 47% of those with a prior-year history of a substance use disorder received UDT, as compared to only 18% of those without such a diagnosis. Given the results of a large 2014 primary care study that found UDT abnormal findings in 30% of samples,[92] it is evident that clinicians too often fail to adhere to the numerous guideline recommendations for use of UDT in patients receiving chronic opioid therapy, thereby putting these patients at a significant risk for harm. These findings suggest that clinicians' behavior with respect to safe prescribing practices and its relationship to the ethical principle of nonmaleficence leaves much room for improvement.

BENEFICENCE

Beneficence refers to the duty of a provider to act in a manner that benefits his or her patient while taking measures to prevent and eliminate potential harms.[4] Widely considered the corollary of nonmaleficence, Gillon[93] has suggested that the relationship between the two principles is better characterized by the need for our efforts to help our patients to be tempered by the imperative not to cause harm in the process. Beneficence is often in obvious contradiction to patient autonomy in the treatment of chronic conditions, as a provider may be focused on avoiding long-term iatrogeneses of the disease and its treatment, which may be inconsistent with the more present-focused preferences of the patient.[94]

The Role of Empathy in Healthcare

Empathy in healthcare has been defined as the "cognitive capacity to understand a patient's needs, an affective sensitivity to a patient's feelings, and a behavioral ability to convey understanding of the patient's feelings."[95(p435)] Empathetic behavior can be considered an aspect of beneficence toward patients.[96] Swindell and colleagues[97] have suggested that empathy is a "tool" for engaging productively with patients, thereby constituting an aspect of "beneficent persuasion." It follows, of course, that beneficent persuasion has the potential to increase patient adherence, as the patient ideally trusts that his or her clinician's directives are well intentioned. However, all too often in pain medicine, our patients feel that our directives are based on our own needs to practice defensive medicine rather than genuine concern for the patients' well-being.[98]

Empathy in Pain Medicine: The Stigma of Dualism

It has been suggested that empathy is disappearing from pain medicine, and perhaps from medicine more broadly. Cohen and colleagues[99] note that there have been, and continue to be, many controversial painful medical conditions (e.g., "railway spine," "occupational neurosis," "whiplash," "nonspecific low back pain," "fibromyalgia syndrome") whose lack of identifiable organic pathology has led to the attribution of psychogenesis as the default interpretation. Cartesian dualism results in stigmatization of patients with chronic, difficult-to-explain pain—not only by society as a whole but by clinicians who invoke the stigma of the "weak mind," which may more reflect lack of understanding of these conditions. Stigmatization tends to be a response to patients (or their conditions) that stand out by appearing or acting differently than the commonly accepted norm.[100] This results in an "us against them" mentality, with negative attributes conferred upon "them."[101] Causing yet further divide is our dichotomization of pain as experienced by the sufferer as being either "good" (eudynia) or "bad" (maldynia).[102] Giordano[103] has astutely noted that although *maldynia* was originally a term used to describe intractable pain, it has devolved to denote "nonpurposiveness." This lack of purpose serves to exacerbate the vulnerability of patients with chronic pain. Recently, Peppin and Schatman[104] addressed the role of terminology in attributions of legitimacy or illegitimacy of chronic pain. Despite pain mechanisms' inability to discriminate between cancer and noncancer pain etiology, these two underlying causes of pain are considered, and accordingly treated, very differently. This difference can be operationalized in our society's willingness to allow opioid analgesia for "cancer pain," while deeming it taboo for those with "noncancer pain."[105]

The tragic result of the antiquated Cartesian model–based stigmatization of patients with chronic pain is what Cohen and his colleagues refer to as "the extinction of empathy"[99] among treating physicians. Empathetic behavior is essential in medicine, as it breeds prosocial, beneficent behaviors, such as compassion.[106] Banja[107] has noted that in order to mitigate the uncomfortable reality of treatment failure, physicians will resort to "stigmatizing, blaming, distrusting, disliking, disagreeing, arguing, denying, rationalizing, or whatever, the objective of a nonempathetic response is to distance and protect the professional from the disturbing stimulus (i.e., the patient's persistent complaints)."[(p1579)] This clearly explains why patients with chronic pain so often feel that their physicians are not particularly enamored with treating them, to say the least.[108]

The Impact of Stigmatization of Patients with Pain

What is the impact of a perceived lack of empathy on adherence among patients with chronic pain? More than a quarter of a century ago, Squier[109] noted the growing trend toward treating clinician–patient relationships as if they were mere business transactions, with an accompanying and unfortunate devolution of the relationship resulting in impaired adherence in the treatment of chronic conditions. Physician empathy has been noted as the "cornerstone" of the concordance model of patient adherence.[110] In a meta-analysis of the relationship between clinician communication and patient adherence to treatment, a significant correlation was found. The authors concluded that empathy was an *essential* element of the clinician–patient relationship.[111] It has been demonstrated that patient-perceived practitioner empathy has improved adherence in a number of conditions and types of treatment, including weight management,[111] oncologic treatment plans,[113] diabetes,[114] control of hemoglobin A1c and low-density lipoprotein cholesterol in diabetics,[115] patient expectations regarding immunomodulatory therapy for multiple sclerosis (which were positively related with continuation of treatment),[116] acceptance of inpatient medical rehabilitation,[117] medication compliance in bipolar disorder,[118] depression,[119] and medication regimens in high-risk tuberculosis.[120] Interestingly, a thorough review of the literature failed to yield any studies of practitioner empathy and its impact on adherence in pain medicine. However, the results of the numerous studies cited here can be extrapolated to patients with chronic pain. It would be difficult to argue that clinician empathy is not beneficent and that the ethical provider should do all that is possible to maintain an empathetic stance toward his or her patients, even (or perhaps especially) with patients that are difficult.

JUSTICE

Justice in medical bioethics is primarily localized to the domain of distributive justice and refers to the fair and equitable distribution of health care resources and services.[4] In regard to adherence, justice should be seen as an extremely relevant issue—particularly in the American healthcare system in which high-quality pain care seems to be becoming progressively more difficult to access. Pain treatment in the form of over-the-counter and prescription drugs in the United States is not a scarce commodity, per se, but *high-quality, safe, and effective comprehensive* pain care has always been limited, and it is becoming increasingly scarce. Should it be reserved only for the most adherent patients? Perhaps this question is best answered by considering the availability of those treatments for which the evidence-bases are strongest.

The Relative Unavailability of Comprehensive Pain Programs

In 2010, a group of pain rehabilitation experts, including a physiatrist, a psychiatrist, a psychologist, a physical therapist, and a biofeedback therapist,[121] reviewed the evidence on rehabilitative treatment of chronic low back pain. They concluded that physical therapy emphasizing graded exercise and psychological treatments such as cognitive behavior therapy and biofeedback constitute the core elements of effective rehabilitation. Although it has been argued that such treatment is most effectively and cost-efficiently provided through comprehensive interdisciplinary chronic pain management programs,[122,123] these programs are now *rarely* available to chronic pain sufferers in the United States outside of the Veterans Administration (VA) healthcare system. In the late-1990s, it was estimated that there were more than 1,000 comprehensive treatment programs in

the United States,[124] but, unfortunately, that number dropped precipi-
tously over the following decade, with only 90 programs remaining in a
late 2012 study.[125] Currently, there are only 55 programs accredited in
the United States by the Commission on Accreditation of Rehabilitation
Facilities, with 19 of the 55 currently in the VA system.[126] Schatman[127,128]
has previously addressed issues of distributive justice associated with the
demise of interdisciplinary pain management in the United States. What
can be concluded is that patients cannot adhere to a treatment paradigm
that is not available to them, through no fault of their own. And when the
unavailable form of treatment itself encourages, reinforces, and demonstrates improved adherence, in contrast to more unidimensional medical
models, that is a big problem. Distributive justice implies inequitable distribution, or preferential treatment. In this case, very few patients with
complex chronic pain conditions are receiving the type of care that has
been demonstrated to be most beneficial and most likely to yield durable
adherence.

The Dearth of Physical Therapists

Physical therapists are integral members of the interdisciplinary (comprehensive) pain care team. Is physical therapy, in particular that emphasizing
graded exercise, of finite or of unlimited supply? In a 2012 study, Zimbelman
and colleagues[129] predicted physical therapist shortages in all 50 states. In a
recent study using stock-and-flow methodology,[130] the authors determined
that the 2010 shortage of 20,000 physical therapists will potentially grow
to as high as 46,000 by 2020. The demand for qualified physical therapists
will likely continue to grow as a result of the Affordable Care Act leading to
greater access to healthcare services by many who previously were unable
to obtain care due to lack of insurance coverage. Clinicians specializing
in pain management are becoming progressively more frustrated in their
efforts to find physical therapists who are trained in chronic pain to treat
their patients. This is not surprising, given findings of a 2015 study[131] that
indicate that American physical therapy students now receive fewer than
four hours of training in exercise training for pain control. Progressively,
physical therapy training programs are emphasizing education in more
technologic approaches that have not been demonstrated to be beneficial
to patients with chronic pain.

Given the growing physical therapist shortage, how does the principle of
distributive justice inform issues of nonadherence in physical therapy? Not
surprisingly, patient adherence has been empirically established as a key

determinant of the success of exercise programs.[132] We opine that patients with chronic pain who are blatantly and persistently nonadherent with their exercise programs do not necessarily have the "right" to what is progressively becoming the "scarce commodity" of high-quality physical therapy. Ideally, nonadherent patients will be referred to a pain psychologist in order to address such nonadherence or, at the minimum, receive counseling from their physicians. Should such efforts be unsuccessful, however, discharge from the treatment program or even the practice is often considered. However, Sciberras and colleagues[133] have noted that nonadherence can be either intentional or unintentional. This raises the question of whether we should treat intentional versus unintentional nonadherence differently. For example, patients with chronic pain are often morbidly depressed,[134] and depression can potentially adversely affect adherence in physical therapy.[135] Should these patients be penalized for their nonadherence in physical therapy if it is due to their depression? This is an ethical dilemma to which there is no clear and absolute answer. However, evaluating for and targeting depression as an incipient cause of poor motivation, energy, or fatigue is a factor that should always be considered before reaching for the "distributive justice" card.

The Other Side of the Coin: Therapist Nonadherence

In addition to patient nonadherence with physical therapy and exercise programs, issues of *therapist* nonadherence should be addressed. Data indicate that physical therapists generally do not implement evidence-based treatment, despite the fact that it is known to improve outcomes and reduce costs.[136,137] If a patient's treatment is less successful due to a failure of a physical therapist to adhere to evidence-based guidelines, this confounds the issue of justice even further. Inadequate treatment can result in patients not realizing functional gains and pain relief or, at a minimum, lengthening the duration of treatment. In such situations, patients are not only unfairly deprived of pain relief but the ability and right to participate in activities in which they should be able to participate. Taking the concern further, if nonevidence-based physical therapy fails to result in functional improvements, a patient may not be able to work—thereby depriving him or her of the right to earn an adequate living and enjoy both the necessities and the luxuries of life to which they would have had access had they received appropriate treatment. This clearly contradicts the principle of "justice." Although we make this argument in regard to physical therapy, the failure of *all* pain treatment professionals to adhere to evidence-based guidelines can potentially have broad, deleterious repercussions

The Role of Clinical Psychologists

Not only is there a diminishing number of physical therapists; there is also a drastic shortage of specifically trained pain psychologists.[58] Bhandari and colleagues[138] have noted that while some doctoral programs offer experiences in pain management, the initial opportunity to specialize as a pain psychologist is usually found in fellowships. However, as postdoctoral fellowships tend to emphasize development of pain research skills, it is apparent that the vast majority of trained pain psychologists are employed on a full-time basis in academic settings. Ironically, our literature search yielded almost 200 hits for "pain psychologist"—almost all of which came from academic medical centers. Accordingly, many academic pain care providers are unaware of this shortage. Our "target patient" is a highly motivated individual with chronic pain whose emotional and/or behavioral issues are interfering with his or her ability to maximize rehabilitative potential, thereby resulting in a lack of physical progress. Yet there are certainly instances in which patients working with pain psychologists are nonadherent. Just as patients with chronic pain may be nonadherent to physical therapists' directives to engage in certain exercises between treatment sessions, psychologists' patients may be nonadherent to our directives to practice self-regulation strategies (e.g., relaxation techniques) that are taught in treatment sessions. Should these patients be discharged, thereby allowing the pain psychologist to take a more motivated patient off his or her waiting list? Can a patient be depressed to the point that working on self-regulation strategies is unrealistic? Again, clear-cut answers to such questions remain elusive.

In terms of *psychologist* nonadherence to guidelines for treatment, we are not aware of the existence of such. A review of the literature indicates the existence of guidelines for the treatment of numerous pain conditions that mention psychological treatment, yet specific psychological treatment guidelines appear to be lacking. Certainly, those treatments falling under the broad rubric of cognitive behavioral therapies and self-regulatory approaches have the strongest evidence bases for psychological intervention for chronic pain[139,140] and are likely the approaches that pain psychologists emphasize. However, if a pain psychologist were to utilize psychoanalytic techniques to treat chronic pain (for which there exists no evidence basis),[141] he or she would be demonstrating nonadherence—particularly if that psychologist had been trained in techniques that have been empirically established as clinically effective.

Finding Balance in the Use of Opioids

The "opioid crisis" of abuse, overdose, and death that the United States has witnessed in recent years has resulted in some believing that the pendulum has swung too far in the direction of fearing opioids, with concerns of[142,143] regulatory sanctions fueled by the media[144] and a resurgent wave of opioid prescribing guidelines (still without strong empirical evidence) causing a "chilling effect." Fears of regulatory sanctions[143] and the publication of numerous opioid prescribing guidelines has resulted in prescribers becoming reluctant to include opioids in their pain management armamentaria, even when other options are not viable or accessible.[145-148] With fewer prescribers, patients with chronic pain are often left without adequate analgesia, experiencing diminished quality of life[149] as well as unnecessary physical limitations. If the number of clinicians willing to prescribe opioids are a scarce resource, then, should access to these clinicians be limited only to the most adherent patients? Again, this is a true "ethical dilemma" (equally and powerfully competing principles) for the clinician facing each individual patient that comes seeking help and for which there is no obvious or easy answer.

CONCLUSIONS

Undoubtedly, many patients suffering from the disease of chronic pain are nonadherent on a variety of levels. However, the same can be said of healthcare providers—particularly those choosing to practice in a nonevidence-based manner. Rather than focusing only on patient adherence, we have chosen to use a framework of principle-based ethics to demonstrate that practitioner adherence is also a glaringly critical issue.

Although we have already left many questions unanswered, we end with yet another, the ethical implications of which are relatively clear. Should not clinicians treating patients with chronic pain do all that they can to maximize their own adherence to model adherent behavior for the patients they treat? The literature suggests that the quality of the clinician–patient relationship has a positive impact not only on patients' emotional responses and physical outcomes but on adherence as well.[150] Patients are more adherent when treated with respect[151] and dignity.[152] We posit that following evidence-based approaches in pain medicine when available, and otherwise acting only in the best interests of the patient (least cost, least risk, highest likelihood of healthy outcomes), is a majestic display of respect and dignity and may indeed lead to greater adherence on the part of our patients. Through fostering greater adherence, clinicians practicing pain medicine honorably may also have the opportunity to demonstrate increased respect for patient autonomy, nonmaleficence, beneficence, and justice—and consequently feel more positive regarding the challenging task that they have chosen to undertake.

The field of pain medicine in the United States has clearly suffered over recent years. To expect our patients to become more adherent *before we do the same* is not necessarily realistic. Somehow, the "extinction of empathy" needs to be reversed. However, at this point, the answer to this dilemma remains elusive.

REFERENCES

1. World Health Organization. *Adherence to Long- Term Therapies: Evidence for Action.* Geneva: World Health Organization; 2003.
2. Nicklas NB, Dunbar M, Wild M. Adherence to pharmacological treatment of non-malignant chronic pain: The role of illness perceptions and medication beliefs. *Psychol Health.* 2010;25:601–615.
3. Solanki DR, Koyyalagunta D, Shah RV, et al. Monitoring opioid adherence in chronic pain patients: assessment of risk of substance misuse. *Pain Physician.* 2011;14:E119–E131.
4. Beauchamp TL, Childress JF. *Principles of Biomedical Ethics,* 5th ed. New York: Oxford University Press, 2001.
5. Kitchener KS. Intuition, critical evaluation and ethical principles: The foundation for ethical decisions in counseling psychology. *Counsel Psychol.* 1984;12:43–55.
6. Rand CS, Sevick MA. Ethics in adherence promotion and monitoring. *Control Clin Trials.* 2000;21(5 Suppl.):S241–S247.
7. Levy AR, Polman RCJ, Borkoles E. Examining the relationship between perceived autonomy support and age in the context of rehabilitation adherence in sport. *Rehabil Psychol.* 2008;53:224–230.
8. Sandman L, Granger BB, Ekman I, Munthe C. Adherence, shared decision-making and patient autonomy. *Med Health Care Philos.* 2012;15:115–127.
9. Cohen MJM, Jasser S, Herron PD, Margolis CG. Ethical perspectives: opioid treatment of chronic pain in the context of addiction. *Clin J Pain.* 2002;18:S99–S107.
10. Falzer PR, Leventhal HL, Peters E, et al. The practitioner proposes a treatment change and the patient declines: what to do next? *Pain Pract.* 2013;13:215–226.
11. Gillon R. Ethics needs principles—four can encompass the rest—and respect for autonomy should be "first among equals." *J Med Ethics.* 2003;29:307–312.

12. Morris GH. Informed consent in psychopharmacology. *Clin J Psychopharmacol.* 2005;25:403–406.

13. Selinger CP. The right to consent: is it absolute? *Br J Med Practitioners.* 2009;2:50–54.

14. Brody H. *Ethical Decisions in Medicine,* 2nd ed. Boston: Little Brown; 1981.

15. Francis CK. Medical ethos and social responsibility in clinical medicine. *J Urban Health.* 2001;78:29–44.

16. Schatman ME. The role of the health insurance industry in perpetuating suboptimal pain management: ethical implications. *Pain Med.* 2011;12:415–426.

17. Schatman ME, Lebovits AH. On the transformation of the "profession" of pain medicine to the "business" of pain medicine: an introduction to a special series. *Pain Med.* 2011;12:403–405.

18. Roter D. The enduring and evolving nature of the patient–physician relationship. *Patient Educ Couns.* 2000;39:5–15.

19. Emanuel EJ, Emanuel LL. Four models of the physician–patient relationship. *JAMA.* 1992;267:2221–2226.

20. Charles C, Gafni A, Whelan T. Shared decision-making in the medical encounter: what does it mean? (or it takes at least two to tango). *Soc Sci Med.* 1997;445:681–692.

21. Schatman ME, Darnall BD. A pendulum swings awry: seeking the middle ground on opioid prescribing for chronic non-cancer pain. *Pain Med.* 2013;14:617–620.

22. Atkinson TJ, Schatman ME, Fudin J. The damage done by the war on opioids: the pendulum has swung too far. *J Pain Res.* 2014;7:265–268.

23. Fudin J, Pratt Cleary J, Schatman ME. The MEDD myth: the impact of pseudoscience on pain research and prescribing guideline development. *J Pain Res.* 2016;Mar 23;9:153–6.

24. Lieber SR, Kim SY, Volk ML. Power and control: contracts and the patient-physician relationship. *Int J Clin Pract.* 2011;65:1214–1217.

25. Gudin JA, Laitman A, Nalamachu S. Opioid related endocrinopathy. *Pain Med.* 2015;16(Suppl. 1):S9–S15.

26. Caplan AL. Informed consent and provider–patient relationships in rehabilitation medicine. *Arch Phys Med Rehabil.* 1988;69:312–317.

27. Hanley EN Jr, Levy JA. Surgical treatment of isthmic lumbosacral spondylolisthesis: analysis of variables influencing results. *Spine* 1989;14:48–50.

28. Basques BA, Bohl DD, Golinvaux NS, Yacob A, Varthi AG, Grauer JN. Factors predictive of increased surgical drain output after anterior cervical discectomy and fusion. *Spine.* 2014;39:728–735.

29. Chapin L, Ward K, Ryken T. Preoperative depression, smoking, and employment status are significant factors in patient satisfaction after lumbar spine surgery. *J Spinal Disord Tech.* 2015 [Epub ahead of print].

30. Parker SL, Mendenhall SK, Godil SS, et al. Incidence of low back pain after lumbar discectomy for herniated disc and its effect on patient-reported outcomes. *Clin Orthop Relat Res.* 2015;473:1988–1999.

31. Weiner BK, Levi BH. The profit motive and spine surgery. *Spine.* 2004;29:2588–2591.

32. Busch AJ, Webber SC, Brachaniec M, et al. Exercise therapy for fibromyalgia. *Curr Pain Headache Rep.* 2011;15:358–367.

33. Dean E, Gormsen Hansen R. Prescribing optimal nutrition and physical activity as "first-line" interventions for best practice management of chronic low-grade

inflammation associated with osteoarthritis: evidence synthesis. *Arthritis.* 2012; 2012:560634.

34. Connelly AE, Tucker AJ, Kott LS, Wright AJ, Duncan AM. Modifiable lifestyle factors are associated with lower pain levels in adults with knee osteoarthritis. *Pain Res Manag.* 2015;20:241–248.

35. Schatman ME, Sullivan J. Whither suffering? The potential impact of tort reform on the emotional and existential healing of traumatically injured chronic pain patients. *Psychol Injury Law.* 2010;3:182–202.

36. Cecil DW. Relational control patterns in physician–patient clinical encounters: continuing the conversation. *Health Comm.* 1998;10(2):125–149.

37. Rehbock T. Limits of autonomy in biomedical ethics? Conceptual clarifications. *Camb Q Healthc Ethics.* 2011;20:524–532.

38. Wicclair MR. Medical paternalism in House M.D. *Med Humanit.* 2008;34: 93–99.

39. McKinstry B. Paternalism and the doctor–patient relationship in general practice. *Br J Gen Pract.* 1992;42:340–342.

40. Giordano J, Schatman, ME. An ethical analysis of crisis in chronic pain care. Part 1: facts, issues, and problems in pain medicine. *Pain Physician.* 2008;11:483–490.

41. Giordano J, Schatman ME. A crisis in chronic pain care: an ethical analysis. Part 2: proposed structure and function of an ethics of pain medicine. *Pain Physician.* 2008;11:589–595.

42. Giordano J, Schatman ME. A crisis in chronic pain care: an ethical analysis. Part 3: toward an integrative, multi-disciplinary pain medicine built around the needs of the patient. *Pain Physician.* 2008;11:771–784.

43. Schwartz DP, Parris WCV. Historical perspectives on pain management. In: Parris WCV, ed. *Contemporary Issues in Chronic Pain Management.* New York: Springer Science + Business Media; 1991:1–8.

44. Breuer B, Pappagallo M, Tai JY, Portenoy RK. U.S. board-certified pain physician practices: uniformity and census data of their locations. *J Pain.* 2007;8:244–250.

45. Cohen M, Quintner J, Buchanan D, Nielsen M, Guy L. Stigmatization of patients with chronic pain: the extinction of empathy. *Pain Med.* 2011;12:1637–1673.

46. Banja J. Empathy in the physician's pain practice: benefits, barriers, and recommendations. *Pain Med.* 2006;7:265–275.

47. Schatman ME. Psychological assessment of maldynic pain: the need for a phenomenological approach. In: Giordano J, ed. *Maldynia: Interdisciplinary Perspectives on the Illness of Chronic Pain.* New York: Informa Healthcare; 2010:157–182.

48. Sullivan MD, Ballantyne J. Must we reduce pain intensity to treat chronic pain? *Pain.* 2016;157:65–69.

49. Ruble J. Off-label prescribing of medications for pain: maintaining optimal care at an intersection of law, public policy, and ethics. *J Pain Palliat Care Pharmacother.* 2012;26:146–152.

50. National Institute on Drug Abuse. Overdose death rates (revised December 2015). Available at https://www.drugabuse.gov/related-topics/trends-statistics/overdose-death-rates. Accessed February 11, 2016.

51. Argoff CE, Kahan M, Sellers EM. Preventing and managing aberrant drug-related behavior in primary care: systematic review of outcomes evidence. *J Opioid Manage.* 2014;10:119–134.

52. Gourlay DL, Heit HA, Almahrezi A. Universal precautions in pain medicine: a rational approach to the treatment of chronic pain. *Pain Med.* 2005;6:107–112.

53. Krebs EE, Ramsey DC, Miloshoff JM, Bair MJ. Primary care monitoring of long-term opioid therapy among veterans with chronic pain. *Pain Med.* 2011;12:740–746.

54. Morasco BJ, Duckart JP, Dobscha SK. Adherence to clinical guidelines for opioid therapy for chronic pain in patients with substance use disorder. *J Gen Intern Med.* 2011;26:965–971.

55. Starrels JL, Becker WC, Weiner MG, Li X, Heo M, Turner BJ. Low use of opioid risk reduction strategies in primary care even for high risk patients with chronic pain. *J Gen Intern Med.* 2011;26:958–964.

56. Morasco BJ, Dobscha SK. Prescription medication misuse and substance use disorder in VA primary care patients with chronic pain. *Gen Hosp Psychiatry* 2008;30:93–99.

57. Sullivan MD, Edlund MJ, Zhang L, Unützer J, Wells KB. Association between mental health disorders, problem drug use, and regular prescription opioid use. *Arch Intern Med.* 2006;166:2087–2093.

58. Darnall BD, Scheman J, Davin S, JW, et al. Pain psychology: a global needs assessment and national call to action. *Pain Med.* 2016 Feb;17(2):250–63.

59. McCracken LM, Gross RT, Aikens J, Carnrike CLM Jr. The assessment of anxiety and fear in persons with chronic pain: a comparison of instruments. *Behav Res Ther.* 1996;34:927–933.

60. Geisser ME, Roth RS, Robinson ME. Assessing depression among persons with chronic pain using the Center for Epidemiological Studies–Depression Scale and the Beck Depression Inventory: a comparative analysis. *Clin J Pain.* 1997;13:163–170.

61. Brown TA, Chorpita BF, Korotitsch W, Barlow DH. Psychometric properties of the Depression Anxiety Stress Scales (DASS) in clinical samples. *Behav Res Ther.* 1997;35:79–89.

62. Sullivan MJ, Stanish WD. Psychologically based occupational rehabilitation: the Pain-Disability Prevention Program. *Clin J Pain.* 2003;19:97–104.

63. Butler SF, Budman SH, Fernandez KC, Fanciullo GJ, Jamison RN. Cross-validation of a screener to predict opioid misuse in chronic pain patients (SOAPP-R). *J Addict Med.* 2009;3:66–73.

64. Passik SD, Weinreb HJ. Managing chronic nonmalignant pain: overcoming obstacles to the use of opioids. *Adv Therapy.* 2000;17(2):70–83.

65. Bell TJ, Panchal SJ, Miaskowski C, Bolge SC, Milanova T, Williamson R. The prevalence, severity, and impact of opioid-induced bowel dysfunction: results of a US and European Patient Survey (PROBE 1). *Pain Med.* 2009;10:35–42.

66. Camilleri M, Drossman DA, Becker G, Webster LR, Davies AN, Mawe GM. Emerging treatments in neurogastroenterology: a multidisciplinary working group consensus statement on opioid-induced constipation. *Neurogastroenterol Motil.* 2014;26:1386–1395.

67. Coyne KS, LoCasale RJ, Datto CJ, Sexton CC, Yeomans K, Tack J. Opioid-induced constipation in patients with chronic noncancer pain in the USA, Canada, Germany, and the UK: descriptive analysis of baseline patient-reported outcomes and retrospective chart review. *Clinicoecon Outcomes Res.* 2014;6:269–281.

68. Iyer S, Davis KL, Candrilli S. Opioid use patterns and health care resource utilization in patients prescribed opioid therapy with and without constipation. *Manag Care.* 2010;19:44–51.

69. Whitman CB, Reid MW, Arnold C, et al. Balancing opioid-induced gastrointestinal side effects with pain management: insights from the online community. *J Opioid Manag.* 2015;11:383–391.

70. Deyo RA, Von Korff M, Duhrkoop D. Opioids for low back pain. *BMJ*. 2015;350:g6380.

71. Katz N, Fanciullo GJ. Role of urine toxicology testing in the management of chronic opioid therapy. *Clin J Pain*. 2002;18(4 Suppl.):S76–S82.

72. Kahan M, Srivastava A, Wilson L, Gourlay D, Midmer D. Misuse of and dependence on opioids: study of chronic pain patients. *Can Fam Physician*. 2006;52:1081–1087.

73. Reisfield GM, Salazar E, Bertholf RL. Rational use and interpretation of urine drug testing in chronic opioid therapy. *Ann Clin Lab Sci*. 2007;37:301–314.

74. Compton P. The role of urine toxicology in chronic opioid analgesic therapy. *Pain Manag Nurs*. 2007;8:166–172.

75. Nafziger AN, Bertino JS Jr. Utility and application of urine drug testing in chronic pain management with opioids. *Clin J Pain*. 2009;25:73–79.

76. Cone EJ, Caplan YH. Urine toxicology testing in chronic pain management. *Postgrad Med*. 2009;121:91–102.

77. Gilbert JW, Wheeler GR, Mick GE, et al. Importance of urine drug testing in the treatment of chronic noncancer pain: implications of recent Medicare policy changes in Kentucky. *Pain Physician*. 2010;13:167–186.

78. Vadivelu N, Chen IL, Kodumudi V, Ortigosa E, Gudin MT. The implications of urine drug testing in pain management. *Curr Drug Saf*. 2010;5:267–270.

79. Christo PJ, Manchikanti L, Ruan X, et al. Urine drug testing in chronic pain. *Pain Physician*. 2011;14:123–143.

80. McCarberg BH1. A critical assessment of opioid treatment adherence using urine drug testing in chronic pain management. *Postgrad Med*. 2011;123:124–131.

81. Jamison RN, Serraillier J, Michna E. Assessment and treatment of abuse risk in opioid prescribing for chronic pain. *Pain Res Treat*. 2011:941808.

82. Atluri S, Akbik H, Sudarshan G. Prevention of opioid abuse in chronic non-cancer pain: an algorithmic, evidence based approach. *Pain Physician*. 2012;15(3 Suppl):ES177–E189.

83. Sehgal N, Manchikanti L, Smith HS. Prescription opioid abuse in chronic pain: a review of opioid abuse predictors and strategies to curb opioid abuse. *Pain Physician*. 2012;15(3 Suppl.):ES67–E92.

84. Gudin JA, Mogali S, Jones JD, Comer SD. Risks, management, and monitoring of combination opioid, benzodiazepines, and/or alcohol use. *Postgrad Med*. 2013;125:115–130.

85. Nuckols TK, Anderson L, Popescu I, et al. Opioid prescribing: a systematic review and critical appraisal of guidelines for chronic pain. *Ann Intern Med*. 2014;160:38–47.

86. Cheung CW, Qiu Q, Choi SW, Moore B, Goucke R, Irwin M. Chronic opioid therapy for chronic non-cancer pain: a review and comparison of treatment guidelines. *Pain Physician*. 2014;17:401–414.

87. Agarin T, Trescot AM, Agarin A, Lesanics D, Decastro C. Reducing opioid analgesic deaths in America: what health providers can do. *Pain Physician*. 2015;18:E307–E322.

88. Sekhon R, Aminjavahery N, Davis CN Jr, Roswarski MJ, Robinette C. Compliance with opioid treatment guidelines for chronic non-cancer pain (CNCP) in primary care at a Veterans Affairs Medical Center (VAMC). *Pain Med*. 2013;14:1548–1556.

89. Khalid L, Liebschutz JM, Xuan Z, et al. Adherence to prescription opioid monitoring guidelines among residents and attending physicians in the primary care setting. *Pain Med*. 2015;16:480–487.

90. Starrels JL, Becker WC, Weiner MG, Li X, Heo M, Turner BJ. Low use of opioid risk reduction strategies in primary care even for high risk patients with chronic pain. *J Gen Intern Med.* 2011;26:958–964.

91. Morasco BJ, Duckart JP, Dobscha SK. Adherence to clinical guidelines for opioid therapy for chronic pain in patients with substance use disorder. *J Gen Intern Med.* 2011;26:965–971.

92. Turner JA, Saunders K, Shortreed SM, et al. Chronic opioid therapy urine drug testing in primary care: prevalence and predictors of aberrant results. *J Gen Intern Med.* 2014;29:1663–1671.

93. Gillon R. Beneficence: doing good for others. *Br Med J.* 1985;291:44–45.

94. Reach G. Patient autonomy in chronic care: solving a paradox. *Patient Prefer Adherence.* 2014;8:15–24.

95. Feighny KM, Monaco M, Arnold L. Empathy training to improve physician–patient communication skills. *Acad Med.* 1995;70:435–436.

96. Bouma HK. Is empathy necessary for the practice of "good" medicine? *Open Ethics J.* 2008;2:1–12.

97. Swindell JS, McGuire AL, Halpern SD. Beneficent persuasion: techniques and ethical guidelines to improve patients' decisions. *Ann Fam Med.* 2010;8:260–264.

98. Payne R, Anderson E, Arnold R, et al. A rose by any other name: pain contracts and agreements. *Am J Bioeth.* 2010;10:5–11.

99. Cohen M, Quintner J, Buchanan D, Nielsen M, Guy L. Stigmatization of patients with chronic pain: the extinction of empathy. *Pain Med.* 2011;12:1637–1643.

100. Link BG, Phelan JC. Conceptualizing stigma. *Annu Rev Sociol.* 2001;27:363–385.

101. Van Rijssen HJ, Schellart AJM, Berkhof M, Anema JR, van der Beek AJ. Stereotyping of medical disability claimants' communication behaviour by physicians: towards more focused education for social insurance physicians. *BMC Public Health.* 2010;10:666.

102. Dickinson BD, Head CA, Gitlow S, Osbahr AJ. Maldynia: Pathophysiology and management of neuropathic and maladaptive pain—a report of the AMA Council on Science and Public Health. *Pain Med.* 2010;11:1635–1653.

103. Giordano J. Maldynia—the illness of chronic pain. In: Giordano J, ed. *Malydnia: Multidisciplinary Perspectives on the Illness of Chronic Pain.* Boca Raton, FL: CRC Press; 2011:1–5.

104. Peppin JF, Schatman ME. Terminology of chronic pain: the need to "level the playing field." *J Pain Res.* 2016;9:23–24.

105. Atkinson TJ, Schatman ME, Fudin J. The damage done by the war on opioids: the pendulum has swung too far. *J Pain Res.* 2014;7:265–268.

106. Davis H. Too early for a neuropsychology of empathy. *Behav Brain Sci.* 2002;25:32–33.

107. Banja JD. Stigmatization, empathy, and the ego depletion hypothesis. *Pain Med.* 2011;12:1579–1580.

108. Upshur CC, Bacigalupe G, Luckmann R. "They don't want anything to do with you": patient views of primary care management of chronic pain. *Pain Med.* 2010;11:1791–1798.

109. Squier RW. A model of empathetic understanding and adherence to treatment regimens in practitioner–patient relationships. *Soc Sci Med.* 1990;30:325–339.

110. Vermeire E, Hearnshaw H, Van Royen P, Denekens J. Patient adherence to treatment: three decades of research. A comprehensive review. *J Clin Pharm Ther.* 2001;26:331–342.

111. Haskard-Zolnierek KB, DiMatteo MR. Physician communication and patient adherence to treatment: a meta-analysis. *Med Care.* 2009;47:826–834.
112. Pollak KI, Østbye T, Alexander SC, et al. Empathy goes a long way in weight loss discussions. *J Fam Pract.* 2007;56:1031–1036.
113. Butow PN, Dunn SM, Tattersall MH, Jones QJ. Computer-based interaction analysis of the cancer consultation. *Br J Cancer.* 1995;71:1115–1121.
114. Mishali M, Sominsky L, Heymann AD. Reducing resistance to diabetes treatment using short narrative interventions. *Fam Pract.* 2010;27:192–197.
115. Hojat M, Louis DZ, Markham FW, Wender R, Rabinowitz C, Gonnella JS. Physicians' empathy and clinical outcomes for diabetic patients. *Acad Med.* 2011;86:359–364.
116. Bischoff C, Schreiber H, Bergmann A. Background information on multiple sclerosis patients stopping ongoing immunomodulatory therapy: a multicenter study in a community-based environment. *J Neurol.* 2012;259:2347–2353.
117. Quaschning K, Körner M, Wirtz M. Analyzing the effects of shared decision-making, empathy and team interaction on patient satisfaction and treatment acceptance in medical rehabilitation using a structural equation modeling approach. *Patient Educ Couns.* 2013;91:167–175.
118. Sylvia LG, Hay A, Ostacher MJ, et al. Association between therapeutic alliance, care satisfaction, and pharmacological adherence in bipolar disorder. *J Clin Psychopharmacol.* 2013;33:343–350.
119. Kaplan JE, Keeley RD, Engel M, Emsermann C, Brody D. Aspects of patient and clinician language predict adherence to antidepressant medication. *J Am Board Fam Med.* 2013;26:409–420.
120. Shimamura T, Taguchi A, Kobayashi S, Nagata S, Magilvy JK, Murashima S. The strategies of Japanese public health nurses in medication support for high-risk tuberculosis patients. *Public Health Nurs.* 2013;30:370–378.
121. Robinson JP, Leo R, Wallach J, McGough E. Schatman ME. Rehabilitative treatment for chronic pain. In: Stannard C, Kalso E, Ballantyne JC, eds. *Evidence-Based Chronic Pain Management.* Oxford: Blackwell; 2010:407–423.
122. Gatchel RJ, Okifuji A. Evidence-based scientific data documenting the treatment and cost-effectiveness of comprehensive pain programs for chronic non-malignant pain. *J Pain* 2006;7:779–793.
123. Turk DC, Swanson K. Efficacy and cost-effectiveness treatment of chronic pain: an analysis and evidence-based synthesis. In: Schatman ME, Campbell A, eds. *Chronic Pain Management: Guidelines for Multidisciplinary Program Development.* New York: Informa Healthcare; 2007:15–38.
124. Anooshian J, Streltzer J, Goebert D. Effectiveness of a psychiatric pain clinic. *Psychosomatics* 1999;40:226–232.
125. Schatman ME. Interdisciplinary chronic pain management: international perspectives. *Pain: Clin Updates.* 2012;20(7):1–5.
126. CARF International. Find an accredited provider. Available at: www.carf.org/prviderSearch.aspx. Accessed February 15, 2016.
127. Schatman ME. The demise of multidisciplinary pain management clinics? *Practical Pain Manage.* 2006;6:30–41.
128. Schatman ME. The demise of the multidisciplinary chronic pain management clinic: bioethical perspectives on providing optimal treatment when ethical principles collide. In: Schatman ME, ed. *Ethical Issues in Chronic Pain Management.* New York: Informa Healthcare; 2007:43–62.

129. Zimbelman JL, Juraschek SP, Zhang X, Lin VW. Physical therapy workforce in the United States: forecasting nationwide shortages. *PM&R*. 2010;2:1021–1029.

130. Landry MD, Hack LM, Coulson E, et al. Workforce projections 2010–2020: annual supply and demand forecasting models for physical therapists across the United States. *Phys Ther*. 2016;96:71–80.

131. Hoeger Bement MK, Sluka KA. The current state of physical therapy pain curricula in the United States: a faculty survey. *J Pain*. 2015;16:144–152.

132. Belza B, Topolski T, Kinne S, Patrick DL, Ramsey SD. Does adherence make a difference? Results from a community-based aquatic exercise program. *Nurs Res*. 2002;51:285–291.

133. Sciberras N, Gregori J, Holt G. The ethical and practical challenge of patient noncompliance in orthopaedic surgery. *J Bone Joint Surg Am*. 2013;95:e61.

134. Magni G, Marchetti M, Moreschi C, Merskey H, Luchini SR. Chronic musculoskeletal pain and depressive symptoms in the nation health and nutrition examination 1: epidemiologic follow-up study. *Pain*. 1993;53:163–168.

135. Jack K, McLean SM, Moffett JK, Gardiner E. Barriers to treatment adherence in physiotherapy outpatient clinics: a systematic review. *Man Ther*. 2010;15:220–228.

136. Ladeira CE, Samuel Cheng M, Hill CJ. Physical therapists' treatment choices for non-specific low back pain in Florida: an electronic survey. *J Man Manip Ther*. 2015;23:109–118.

137. Roberts ET, DuGoff EH, Heins SE, et al. Evaluating clinical practice guidelines based on their association with return to work in administrative claims. *Health Serv Res*. 2016;51(3):953–980.

138. Bhandari R, Kao G, Logan DE. Pediatric pain psychology fellowship training: current trends in the USA and future goals. *Pediatr Pain Letter*. 2014;16:22–28.

139. Hoffman BM, Papas RK, Chatkoff DK, Kerns RD. Meta-analysis of psychological interventions for chronic low back pain. *Health Psychol*. 2007;26:1–9.

140. Kerns RD, Sellinger J, Goodin BR. Psychological treatment of chronic pain. *Annu Rev Clin Psychol*. 2011;7:411–434.

141. Csaszar-Nagy N, Bagdi P, Stoll D, Szoke. Pain and psychotherapy, in the light of evidence of psychological treatment methods of chronic pain based on evidence. *J Psychol Psychother*. 2014;4:145.

142. Schatman ME, Darnall BD. A pendulum swings awry: seeking the middle ground on opioid prescribing for chronic non-cancer pain. *Pain Med*. 2013;14:617–620.

143. Atkinson TJ, Schatman ME, Fudin J. The damage done by the war on opioids: the pendulum has swung too far. *J Pain Res*. 2014;7:265–268.

144. Schatman ME. The American chronic pain crisis and the media: about time to get it right? *J Pain Res*. 2015;8:885–887.

145. Anson P. Death rate from painkiller overdoses drops in Washington State. *National Pain Report*, Jan 28, 2013. Available at http://nationalpainreport.com/death-rate-from-painkiller-overdoses-drops-in-washington-state-8818418.html. Accessed February 28, 2016.

146. McCarberg B. Washington State opioid prescribing guidelines. *Pain Med*. 2015;16:1455–1456.

147. Ruan X, Chiravuri S. The predicament of the undertreatment of chronic pain and prescription opioid epidemic. *Analg Resusc: Curr Res*. 2015;4:1.

148. van Gunten CF. The pendulum swings for opioid prescribing. *J Palliat Med*. 2016 Apr;19(4):348.

149. Berens M, Armstrong K. New state law leaves patients in pain. *Seattle Times*, April 7, 2015. Available at http://seattletimes.com/html/localnews/2016994769_silent12.html. Accessed February 28, 2016.

150. Haynes RB, McDonald HP, Garg AX. Helping patients follow prescribed treatment: clinical applications. *JAMA*. 2002;288:2880–2883.

151. Charon R. The patient-physician relationship: narrative medicine: a model for empathy, reflection, profession, and trust. *JAMA*. 2001;286:1897–1902.

152. Beach MC, Sugarman J, Johnson RL, Arbelaez JJ, Duggan PS, Cooper LA. Do patients treated with dignity report higher satisfaction, adherence, and receipt of preventive care? *Ann Fam Med*. 2005;3:331–338.

INDEX

Page references followed by *f*'s , *t*'s, or *b*'s indicate figures, tables, or boxes respectively.

Morasco, B. J., 145, 165
MORE (Mindfulness-Oriented Recovery
　Enhancement), 50
motivation. *See* patient motivation
motivational interviewing (MI)
　ACT and, 21
　empathy and, 14
　healthcare provider–patient
　　relationship, 104–105
motivational models
　COM-B, 14–15
　goal of, 88
multimodal pain care model, 133

Narcotics Anonymous, 147
National Heart, Lung and Blood
　Institute of the National Institutes
　of Health, 98
National Institute for Health and Care
　Excellence (NICE), 99
natural opioids, 64t
necessary redundancy, viii
Necessity-Concerns Framework, 12–13
negative affect
　opioid craving and, 36
　prescription opioid misuse and, 35
Nelson, C., 22
neurocognitive deficits (socioecological
　model of adherence), 91–92
Newman, M. G., 151
NICE (National Institute for Health and
　Care Excellence), 99
NM-ASSIST (Alcohol, Smoking, and
　Substance Involvement Screening
　Test), 45–46
nonadherence
　chronic pain management, 8–11
　factors affecting, 2
　factors associated with, 33–39
　incidence of, 2–3
　managing patients at risk of, 49–51
　monitoring, 41–46
　screening for patients at risk of, 39–41
noncompliance
　defined, 1–2
　interventions to improve
　　adherence, 49–51
nonmaleficence, 163–165
　monitoring four A's of pain medicine,
　　164–165

overview, 163
psychological assessment of risk of
　substance misuse/abuse, 163–164
nonopioid medications, 36–39
　headache medications, 38–39
　overview, 36–37
　role of UDT in nonopioid-using
　　patients, 73
　sedative-hypnotics, 37–38
nonspecific low back pain, 166
nonsteroidal anti-inflammatory drugs
　(NSAIDs), 36, 37

obesity. *See also* weight loss and physical
　activity
　BMI and, 84
　fibromyalgia and, 85
　low back pain and, 99
　obesogenic environment, 98
　social networks and, 97
*Obesity: Identification, Assessment and
　Management* guideline, 99
Obesity Society, 98
OCC (Opioid Compliance Checklist), 42,
　43t, 48
occupational neurosis, 166
oligoanalgesia, 164
Open process (PF model), 19f, 20
operant conditioning (socioecological
　model of adherence), 93
opiates. *See also* opioids
　cross-reacting drug, 65t
　drug time in urine, 79t
　sources of opioid analgesics, 64t
Opioid Compliance Checklist (OCC), 42,
　43t, 48
opioid contracts, 146–147
opioid craving, 36
opioid receptors, 33
Opioid Risk Tool (ORT), 39, 40t, 41, 139
opioids, 33–36. *See also* opiates
　detoxification, 49
　drug panel testing, 67t–68t
　finding balance in use of, 172
　metabolism of, 72f
　overview, 33–34
　risk factors for prescription misuse
　　and addiction, 34–36
　subjective effects, 37
opioid therapy agreements, 47–48